without the | quick
the | and easy
calories | Justine Pattison

For John, Jess and Emily

Also in the *Without the Calories* series

Takeaway Favourites Without the Calories

Comfort Food Without the Calories

Pasta and Rice Without the Calories

One Pot Without the Calories

Cakes, Cookies and Bread Without the Calories

7   1|8   1|9   2|0   2|1   2|2   2|3   2|4   2|5   2|6   2

without the calories | quick and easy

Justine Pattison

Low-calorie recipes, cheats and
ideas for every day

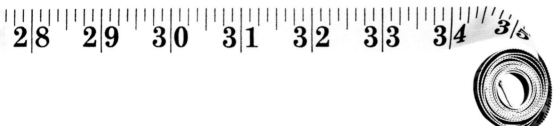

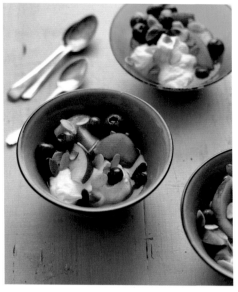

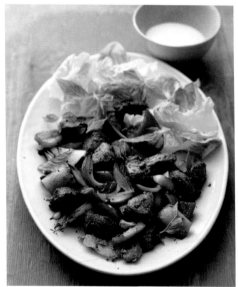

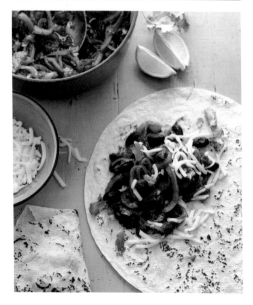

contents

introduction

MY STORY

I struggled with my weight for years. After being a skinny child and teenager, I piled on the weight during my last years of school and went into my twenties feeling fat and frumpy. A career as a cookery writer and food stylist has helped me understand good food but because my kitchen is always overflowing with great things to eat, temptation is never far away. My weight yo-yoed for twenty years and at my heaviest I weighed more than 15 stone.

A few years ago, I worked on the hit TV series *You Are What You Eat* – I put together those groaning tables of bad food. I also had the chance to work with the contributors on the show, guiding them through the dieting process and helping them discover a whole new way of eating and cooking. Having been overweight myself, I became passionate about helping people lose weight.

Since then, I've worked as a food consultant on many of the weight-loss shows you've seen on TV, and written diet plans and recipes for best-selling books, newspapers and magazines. I'm so proud that thousands of people have successfully followed my way of cooking and lost weight.

This book, and the others in the *Without the Calories* series, are ideal for anyone who wants to lose weight while leading a normal life. Cooking my way will help you sustain a happy, healthy weight loss. That's what it's all about: you don't have to be stick thin, but you deserve to feel good about yourself. My *Without the Calories* recipes will help you reach your goal.

ABOUT THIS BOOK

When you are trying to lose weight, cooking instead of relying on convenience foods will help you keep a really close eye on your calories. But if you aren't a confident cook or have very little time to spend in the kitchen, you'll need a collection of quick and easy recipes that can be rustled up in minutes.

In this book, I've created a variety of speedy recipes that shouldn't take more than 45 minutes from start to finish. Most of the recipes take under 30 minutes, but I've tried to be realistic about the time they could take. Recipes that need freezing or marinating may take a little longer, but the preparation time is usually incredibly quick. I've reworked the ingredients to reduce the calories, while still trying hard to keep all the flavour and appetite appeal, helping you lose weight in the most delicious and simple way possible.

I'm not going to make rash promises about how many pounds you will shed, but I do know that when it comes to losing weight, finding foods that give you pleasure and fit into your lifestyle are the key to success. When you eat well without obsessing over rapid weight loss, it's easier to relax and lose what you need to comfortably – and safely.

To help everyone enjoy these dishes, I've used easy-to-find ingredients and given clear, simple cooking instructions. There's lots of freezer information included, so you know which dishes you can store safely for another day.

If you're already following a diet plan, you'll find additional nutritional information at the back of the book that'll help you work my recipes into your week. And, if you're stuck for inspiration and have a few pounds to lose, try my 123 Plan. It couldn't be easier.

USING THE 123 PLAN

If you're not following a diet regime at the moment and want a great kick-start, try my 123 Plan for a few weeks. I've tried to make it really easy, and you don't need to do too much adding up. Just pick one recipe from any section to bring your daily intake to between 900 and 1,200 calories. Add an *essential extra* 300 calories a day and you'll be on your way to a healthy, sustainable weight loss of between 2–3lbs a week.

ONE
up to 300 calories

TWO
300–400 calories

THREE
400–500 calories

YOUR ESSENTIAL EXTRAS

These extra 300 calories can be made up of accompaniments, such as potatoes, rice and pasta, as well as snacks or treats; there are suggestions and serving sizes on page 180. You'll also find recipes that contain under 200 calories a portion, which can be included as part of your essential extras. As long as your extras don't exceed 300 calories a day, you'll be on track.

WHEN TO EAT

The 123 Plan is flexible, so if you find you fancy a **ONE** or **TWO** recipe rather than a **THREE** as your third meal of the day, just add enough calories to bring it into the right range. Don't worry if the calculations aren't absolutely accurate – a difference of 25 or less calories per serving won't affect your weekly allowance.

You don't have to eat your lightest meal for breakfast and the most calorific meal late in the day – in fact, the opposite often works best. I tend to eat my largest meal at lunchtime if I can, and have a lighter meal in the evening, but work with what suits you and your family best.

If you want to add your own favourite meals into the plan, just make sure they are within the recommended calorie boundaries and calculate accordingly. (You may find this useful when planning breakfast especially.)

DON'T RUSH IT

Weight tends to be gained over time, and losing it gradually will make the process easier and help give your body, especially your skin, time to adapt. You're more likely to get into positive, enjoyable long-term cooking and eating habits this way too.

WHAT IS A CALORIE?

Put simply, a calorie is a unit of energy contained within food and drink which our bodies burn as fuel. Different foods contain varying amounts of calories and if more calories are consumed than the body needs, the excess will be stored as fat. To lose weight, we need to eat less or use more energy by increasing our activity – and ideally both!

I've provided the calorie content of a single serving of each dish. In my experience, most people will lose at least 2lb a week by consuming around 1,200–1,500 calories a day, but it's always best to check with your GP before you start a new regime. Everyone is different and, especially if you have several stones to lose, you'll need some personalised advice. The calories contained in each recipe have been calculated as accurately as possible, but could vary a little depending on your ingredients.

A few wayward calories here and there won't make any difference to your overall weight loss.

If you have a couple of days of eating more than 1,400 calories, try to eat closer to 1,100 for the next few days. Over a week, things will even out.

My recipes strike a balance between eating and cooking well and reducing calories, and I've tried them all as part of my own way of enjoying food without putting on excess weight. Even if you don't need to lose weight, I hope you enjoy cooking from my books simply because you like the recipes.

SECRETS OF SUCCESS

The serving sizes that I've recommended form the basis of the nutritional information on page 182, and if you eat any more, you may find losing weight takes longer. If you're cooking for anyone who doesn't need to watch their calorie intake, simply increase their servings and offer plenty of accompaniments.

The right portion size also holds the key to maintaining your weight loss. Use this opportunity to get used to smaller servings. Work out exactly how much food your body needs to maintain the shape that makes you feel great. That way, even when counting calories feels like a distant memory, you'll remain in control of your eating habits.

Stick to lean protein (which will help you feel fuller for longer) and vegetables and avoid high-fat, high-sugar snacks and confectionery. Be aware that alcohol is packed with empty calories and could weaken your resolve. Starchy carbs such as pasta, rice, potatoes and bread are kept to a minimum because I've found that, combined with eating lots of veg and good protein, this leads to more sustainable weight loss. There's no need to avoid dairy products such as cheese and cream, although they tend to be high in fat and calories. You can swap the high-fat versions for reduced-fat ones, or use less.

Ditch heavily processed foods and you will feel so much better. Switching to more natural ingredients will help your body work with you.

If you don't cook often, try a few of my recipes and see how easy they can be.

Most recipes here form the main part of each meal, so there's room to have your plate half-filled with freshly cooked vegetables or a colourful, crunchy salad. This will help fill you up, and boost your intake of vitamins and minerals.

Make sure you drink enough fluids, especially water – around 2 litres is ideal. Staying hydrated will help you lose weight more comfortably, and it's important when you exercise too.

IN THE KITCHEN

Pick up some electronic kitchen scales and a set of measuring spoons if you don't already have them. Both will probably cost less than a takeaway meal for two, and will help ensure good results.

Invest, if you can, in a large, deep non-stick frying pan and a medium non-stick saucepan. The non-stick coating means that you will need less oil to cook, and a frying pan with a wide base and deep sides can double as a wok.

I use oil and butter sparingly, and use a calorie-controlled spray oil for frying. I also keep a jam jar containing a little sunflower oil and a heatproof pastry brush to hand for greasing pans lightly before frying.

STICK WITH IT

Shifting your eating habits and trying to lose weight is not easy, especially if you have been eating the same way for many years. But it isn't too late. You may never have the perfect body, but you can have one that, fuelled by really good food, makes you feel happy and healthy. For more information and menu plans visit www.justinepattison.co.uk.

Enjoy!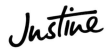

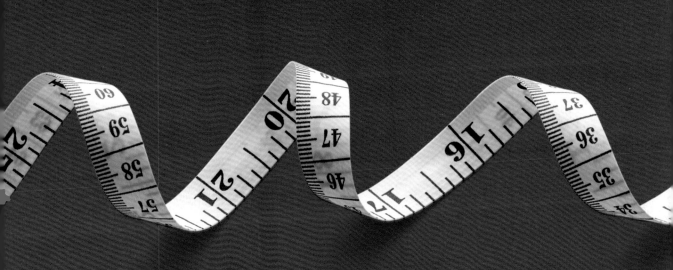

breakfast
and brunch

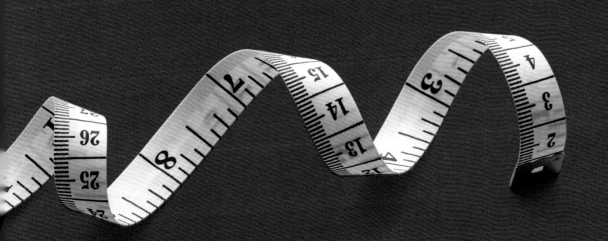

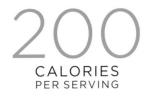

200
CALORIES
PER SERVING

boiled eggs with asparagus soldiers

SERVES 2
PREP: 2 MINUTES
COOK: 10 MINUTES

4 fridge-cold eggs
200g slender asparagus
  spears
flaked sea salt
ground black pepper

Boiled eggs make a great breakfast and easy snack. These are served with freshly cooked asparagus spears instead of a slice of buttered toast for dipping, which will reduce the calories by around 100 per serving. If you only fancy one egg, knock off 80 calories for each serving.

Half fill a small saucepan with water and bring it to the boil. Gently add the eggs to the water with a slotted spoon and return to the boil. (If the eggs are added too roughly, the shells could crack.) Cook for 7 minutes for a soft boiled egg taken from the fridge. (Cook for about 5 minutes if your eggs are at room temperature.)

While the eggs are cooking, fill a wide-based saucepan a third full with water and bring to a simmer. Trim the ends off the asparagus and cook the spears for 2–3 minutes (depending on thickness) or until just tender. Lift out with tongs and divide between two mugs or pots.

Put the eggs in egg cups and place on small plates. Cut off the tops. Serve with the warm asparagus for dipping and a little salt and pepper.

Boiled eggs and toast soldiers: Cook the eggs in exactly the same way as above. Serve each one with a medium slice of wholegrain toast, spread with ½ teaspoon of softened butter. Serves 2. Calories per serving: 267.

Poached egg on toast: Half fill a small pan with water and bring to the boil. Crack an egg into a bowl. Turn the heat down so the water is bubbling gently. Stir the water with a spoon and gently add the egg. Cook for about 2½ minutes, or until the white of the egg is no longer clear but the yolk remains soft. Toast a medium slice of wholemeal bread. Spread ½ teaspoon butter lightly over the toast. Using a slotted spoon, scoop the egg out of the water, drain off any excess water and pop the egg on top of the toast. Top with salt, ground black pepper and some Worcestershire sauce. Serves 1. Calories per serving: 193

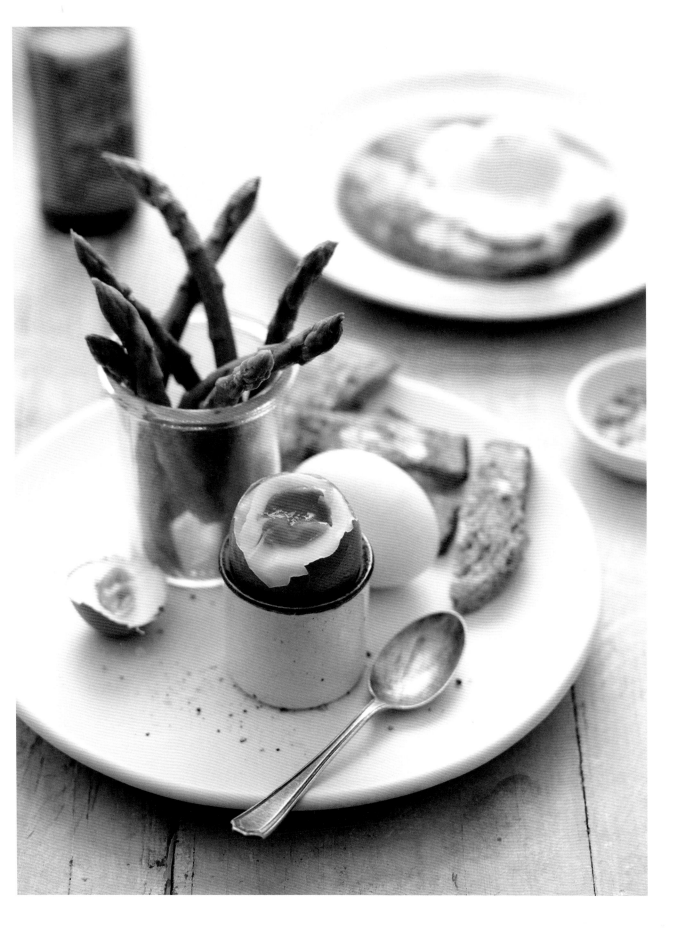

breakfast smoothie

SERVES 1
PREP: 5 MINUTES

1 banana, peeled and sliced
150g strawberries,
  hulled and halved
150ml well-chilled
  semi-skimmed milk
  (or orange juice)
2 tbsp rolled oats,
  (about 15g)

Tip: You can make this smoothie with frozen sliced strawberries or mixed frozen berries if you prefer. Don't forget to use a blender designed to crush ice.

Smoothies make a handy breakfast when time is short and this combination is one of my favourites. Adding a few oats to the mix makes it more filling, but you can leave them out if you prefer. Made with orange juice instead of semi-skimmed milk it will contain 20 fewer calories. For a really light start to the day, try the warm spiced grapefruit (see below).

Put all the ingredients in a blender or food processor and blitz until as smooth as possible. Pour into a tall glass and serve.

Warm spiced grapefruit: Preheat the grill to its hottest setting. Cut a grapefruit in half and slice between each segment with a grapefruit knife or the tip of a vegetable knife. Place on a grill pan, cut side up. Sprinkle with 1 teaspoon sugar tossed with a good pinch of ground mixed spice. Grill for 4–5 minutes or until the grapefruit is warm and the sugar has dissolved. Serves 2. Calories per serving: 32

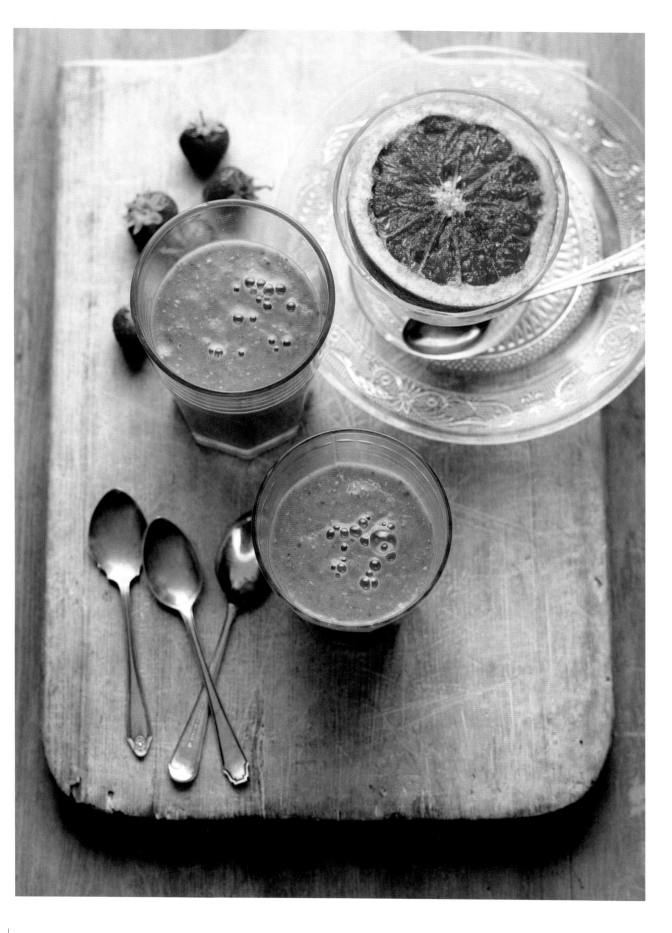

179
CALORIES
PER SERVING

yoghurt pot pancakes

SERVES 4
PREP: 5 MINUTES
COOK: 15 MINUTES

150g pot of fat-free
    natural yoghurt
150ml semi-skimmed milk
100g plain flour
2 eggs
oil, for spraying or brushing
1 lemon, cut into wedges
2 tsp caster sugar

Freeze the cooled pancakes
in a stack, interleaved with
baking parchment, and put
them in a freezer bag.
Freeze for up to 1 month.
Reheat from frozen in a dry
non-stick frying pan for
1 minute, turning frequently
over a medium heat or on
a plate in the microwave
for a few seconds.

This is a brilliantly quick way to prepare pancakes and one
that keeps the kitchen tidy as you only need a bowl, a whisk
and a frying pan to make them. Any leftover pancakes can
be frozen and then reheated in the microwave.

Tip the yoghurt into a bowl then fill the empty pot with semi-
skimmed milk and pour over the top. Refill with plain flour and
sprinkle the flour into the bowl. Break both eggs into the bowl
and beat with a metal whisk until smooth.

Spray or brush a medium non-stick frying pan (with a base
around 19cm wide) with oil and place over a medium-high heat.
Add 3–4 spoonfuls (or a ladleful) of the batter and tilt the pan
to allow the mixture to spread across the pan in a thin layer.

Cook for 2 minutes until set and beginning to lift at the side,
then carefully turn over and cook on the other side for a further
1–2 minutes until lightly browned. Use a palette knife or spatula
to loosen and turn the pancake. Repeat until all the mixture has
been used. If the batter becomes too thick to spread easily,
simply whisk in a little extra milk.

Pile the pancakes onto plates and serve warm with lemon
wedges and sugar.

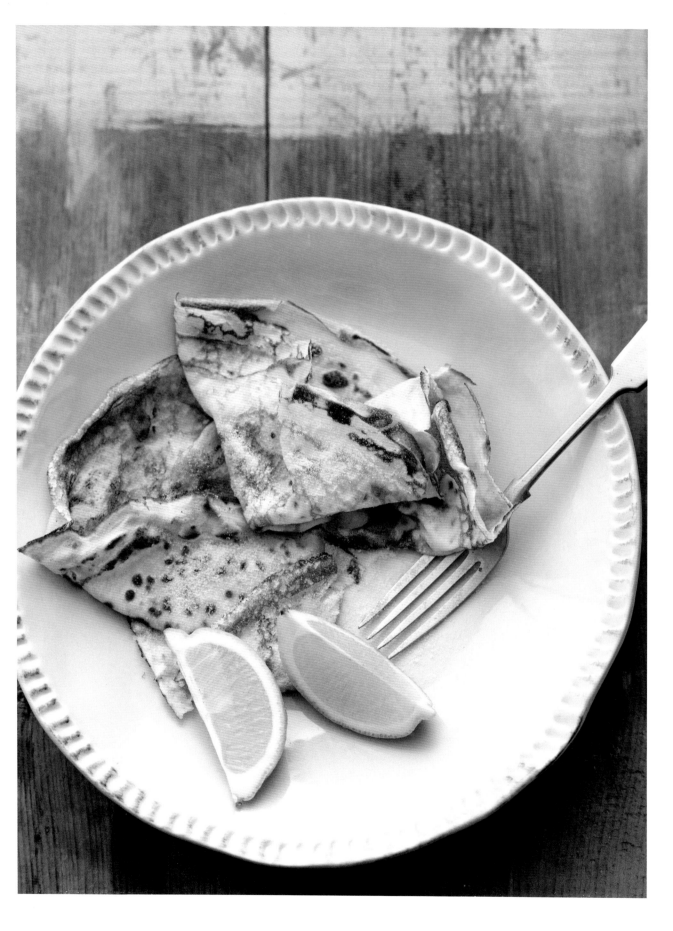

70
CALORIES
PER SERVING

five-minute nectarines with vanilla and star anise

SERVES 4

PREP: 5 MINUTES

COOK: 5 MINUTES

2 ripe nectarines or peaches
2 tbsp cold water
2 star anise
½ tsp vanilla extract or
    vanilla bean paste
200g fat-free Greek-style
    yoghurt
100g fresh blueberries
10g toasted flaked almonds
    (optional)

Tip: To cook the nectarines
in a conventional oven,
place the wedges in a
small ovenproof dish with
2 tablespoons of cold water,
the star anise and vanilla,
cover with foil and bake in
a preheated oven at 200°C/
Fan 180°C/Gas 6 for 20–25
minutes or until softened.

I love poached fruit and it makes a convenient breakfast or dessert, served warm or cold with fat-free yoghurt. You can bake it in the oven, but a quick blast in the microwave gives the same result.

Cut the nectarines into wedges by slicing around the stone in each fruit carefully with a small knife. Put the wedges in a microwave-proof bowl and stir in 2 tablespoons of cold water, the star anise and vanilla.

Cover and cook on the highest setting for 3–5 minutes or until the fruit is soft. Microwave wattages vary, so check every minute to see how the fruit is progressing.

Serve the nectarines with the yoghurt, blueberries and a sprinkling of flaked almonds if you like. (Add an extra 16 calories for each teaspoon of almonds you use.)

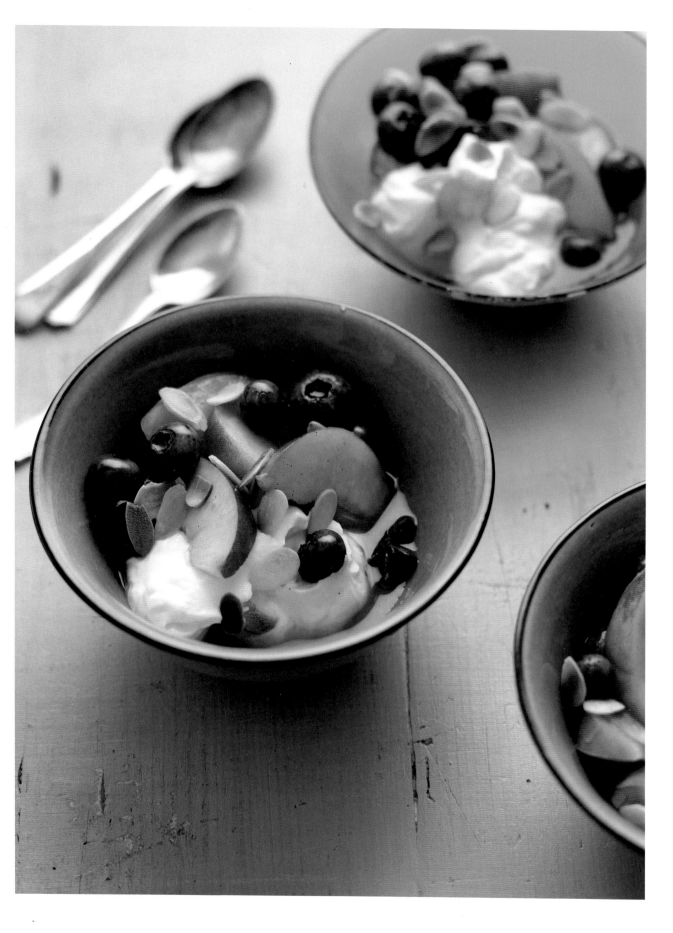

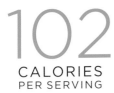

crushed berry layered yoghurt

SERVES 5
PREP: 10 MINUTES

500g fresh (or frozen and
  thawed) mixed berries,
  such as strawberries,
  raspberries, redcurrants
  and blueberries
1–2 tbsp caster sugar
500ml fat-free natural
  yoghurt
½ tsp vanilla extract or
  vanilla bean paste

A stash of these little pots in the fridge means there is never an excuse to miss breakfast. They are easy to transport and make a good snack or dessert too. Use thawed frozen berries instead of fresh if you like and adjust the sweetening to taste, bearing in mind that 1 teaspoon of caster sugar contains around 16 calories. Adding vanilla bean paste to the yoghurt will make it sweeter too.

Hull and cut the strawberries into quarters. Put all the berries in a bowl and mash lightly with 1 tablespoon of the sugar. (Depending on your choice of berries, you may need to add a little more sugar to taste.) Mix the yoghurt with the vanilla.

Spoon the berries into small rubber-seal jars or clean jam jars, layering with the vanilla yoghurt. Cover and seal. Keep chilled and eat within 3 days.

Cherry and chocolate chip muesli: Put 250g porridge oats (not jumbo) and 100g unsweetened puffed rice in a large rubber-sealed jar or plastic food container. Add 40g unsweetened coconut chips or flakes, 40g plain chocolate chips and 75g dried cherries. Mix well. Serve 50g portions of the muesli for breakfast with semi-skimmed milk or low-fat natural yoghurt and some fresh berries if you like.
Serves 12. Calories per serving: 143

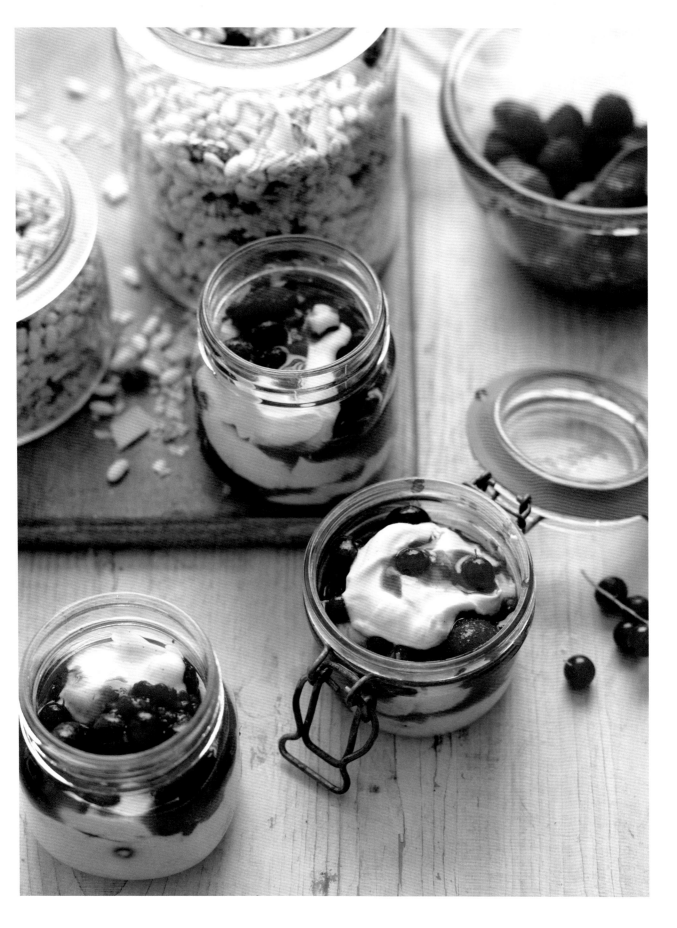

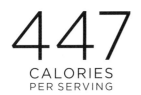

447
CALORIES
PER SERVING

french toast with banana

SERVES 2
PREP: 5 MINUTES
COOK: 2–3 MINUTES

2 eggs
4 slices fruit loaf
  (about 40g each)
10g butter
2 tsp sunflower oil
1 banana, peeled and sliced
50g fresh raspberries
2 tsp maple syrup

French toast, also known in our household as eggy bread, is a delicious breakfast for all the family. You don't need any particular cooking skills to prepare it and it makes a lovely treat at the weekend. The calories are a little higher than in some other breakfasts, but as long as you keep an eye on your daily allowance, you will still lose weight. If you use medium slices of plain white bread from a small loaf, instead of the fruit loaf, you can knock off around 40 calories per serving.

Whisk the eggs in a medium bowl with a metal whisk. Melt half the butter with half the oil in a large non-stick frying pan over a medium heat.

Place two slices of the bread in the whisked egg. Turn the bread until lightly soaked with the egg and put in the frying pan.

Fry the bread for about 1 minute until lightly browned. Using tongs, turn the bread over and cook the other side for a further minute until crisp and golden brown. Put on one large warmed plate or platter. Cook the remaining bread in exactly the same way.

Top the French toast with sliced banana and raspberries. Drizzle with a little maple syrup if you like and serve immediately.

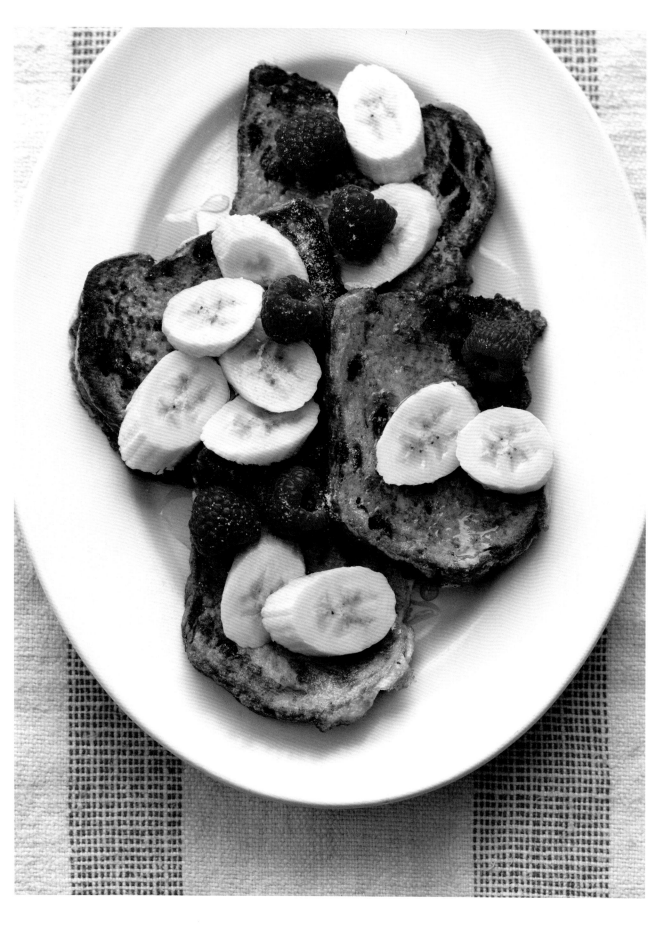

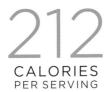

212
CALORIES
PER SERVING

tomatoes on toasted sourdough

SERVES 2
PREP: 5 MINUTES
COOK: 5 MINUTES

2 large ripe tomatoes,
   roughly chopped
1 tsp red wine vinegar
   or sherry vinegar
4 thin slices sourdough
   bread (each about 35g)
½ garlic clove
1 tsp extra virgin olive oil
flaked sea salt
ground black pepper

This makes a fantastic breakfast served with a strong cup of coffee. It's best eaten when the weather is hot and the tomatoes are very ripe. Slicing the sourdough very thinly makes the serving size look generous but keeps the calories low. Serve as a snack or light supper too.

Mix the tomatoes with the vinegar, a good pinch of salt and lots of ground black pepper.

Toast the bread or cook it on a hot griddle until lightly browned. Rub 1 side of each piece of toast with the garlic then put the toast on a plate.

Top with the tomatoes, dribble with the oil and serve.

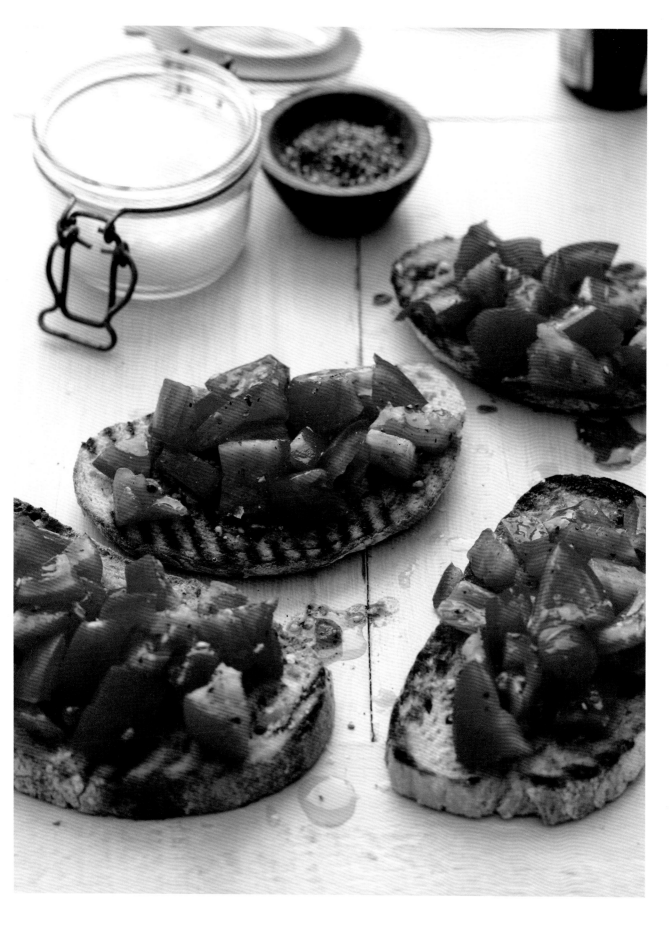

275

scrambled egg with bacon

SERVES 2
PREP: 5 MINUTES
COOK: 5 MINUTES

2 rashers smoked back
    bacon (about 65g)
oil, for spraying or brushing
15g butter
4 eggs
flaked sea salt
ground black pepper

TO SERVE
2 toasted crumpets or
    2 medium slices
    wholemeal bread
fresh cress, to garnish
    (optional)

I always cook my scrambled egg slowly over a low heat to ensure it tastes rich and creamy. Delicious served with smoked bacon on a toasted crumpet or, for roughly 20 calories less, a medium slice of wholemeal toast works just as well. Perfect for a weekend brunch.

Trim any visible fat off the bacon. Heat the oil in a large non-stick frying pan over a medium-high heat. Add the bacon and cook for 2 minutes on each side until lightly browned.

Meanwhile, melt the butter in a medium non-stick saucepan. Beat the eggs in a bowl with a metal whisk until smooth and season with salt and pepper.

Tip the eggs into the saucepan and cook over a low heat for 2 minutes, stirring regularly until lightly set.

Divide the egg between warmed plates and top with the bacon and some cress. Serve immediately with toasted crumpets or sliced wholemeal bread.

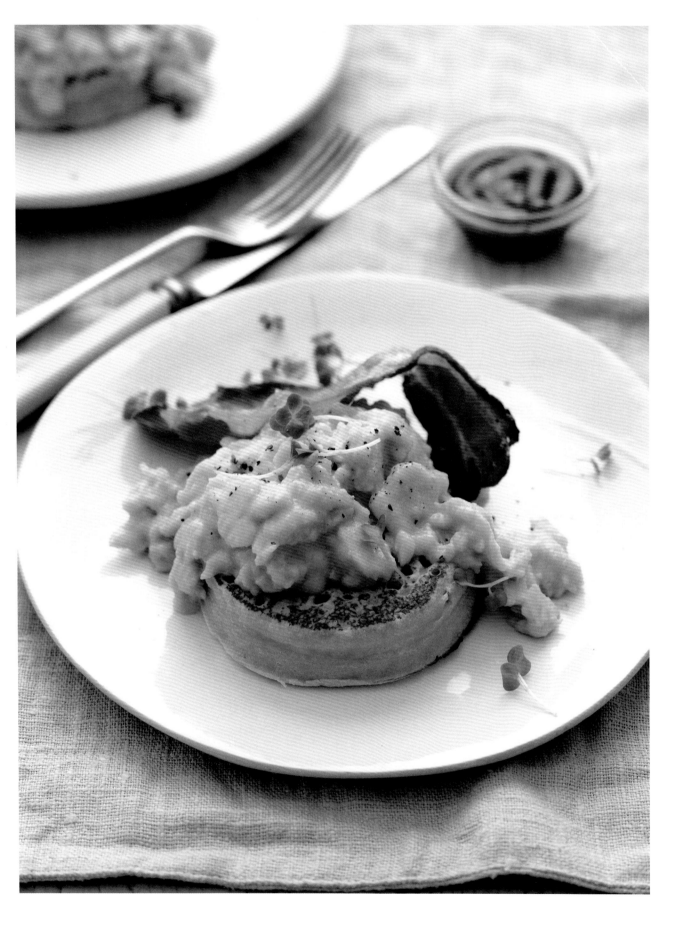

304 CALORIES PER SERVING

mexican breakfast

SERVES 4
PREP: 5 MINUTES
COOK: 15 MINUTES

oil, for spraying or brushing
1 medium red onion,
    thinly sliced
1 yellow pepper, deseeded
    and thinly sliced
½–1 tsp hot smoked paprika,
    depending on taste
400g can chopped
    tomatoes with herbs
400g can red kidney beans,
    drained and rinsed
2 tbsp tomato purée
15g fresh coriander, leaves
    roughly chopped, plus
    extra to garnish
4 very fresh fridge-cold
    eggs
40g ready-grated
    mozzarella or half-fat
    Cheddar (optional)
4 mini flour tortilla wraps
    (each about 30g)
ground black pepper
lime wedges, to serve

I love this spicy start to a lazy weekend and it makes a wonderful lunch or supper dish too. Choose mini flour tortilla wraps – often sold for children's lunch boxes – to serve alongside, as they contain around 90 calories each, about half the calories of a large one.

Spray or brush a large non-stick frying pan with oil. Add the onion and pepper and fry gently for 3–4 minutes until lightly browned. Stir in the paprika and cook for a few seconds more. Tip the tomatoes and kidney beans into the pan and add the tomato purée. Bring to a gentle simmer and cook for 5 minutes, stirring occasionally until thick. Stir in the coriander.

Make a hole in the tomato mixture and break an egg into it. Repeat with the other eggs. Season the eggs with black pepper, cover the pan with a lid or large piece of foil and cook for 4–5 minutes until the egg whites have set and the yolks are hot but runny. If adding the cheese, sprinkle it over the eggs after the first couple of minutes so it has time to melt. Scatter more coriander over the top if you like.

Meanwhile, heat the tortillas in the microwave or a moderate oven according to the packet instructions. Take the eggs and beans to the table and serve with the warm tortillas and lime wedges for squeezing.

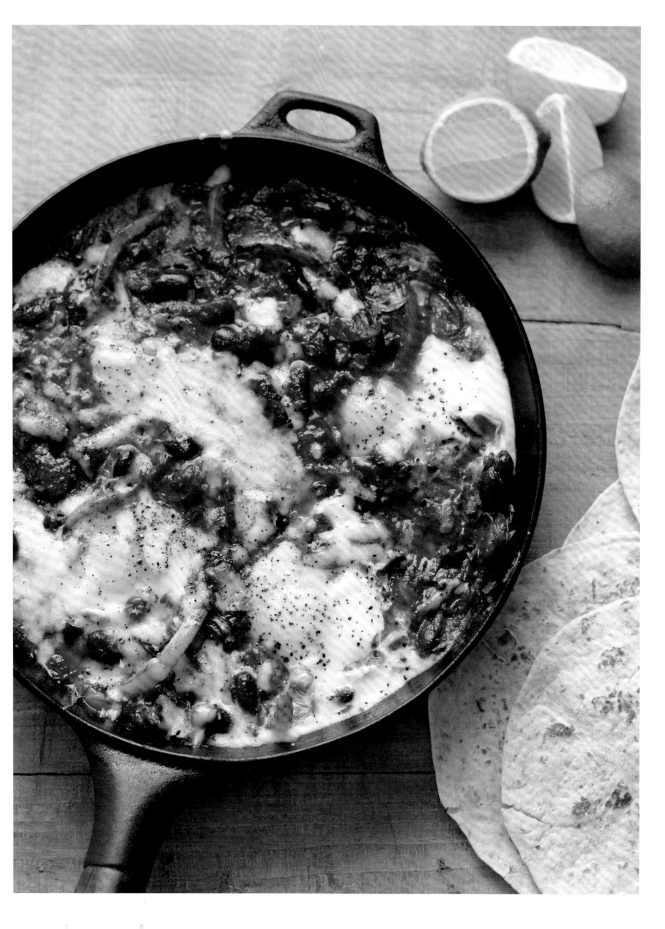

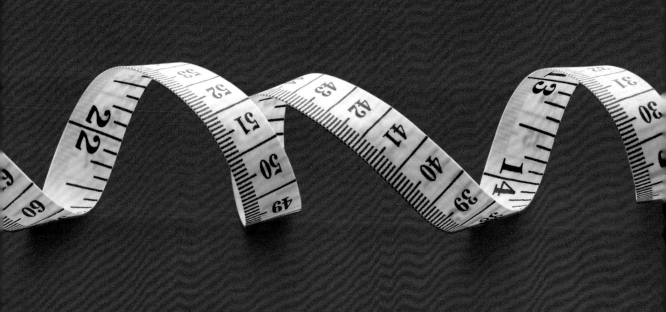

chicken
and turkey

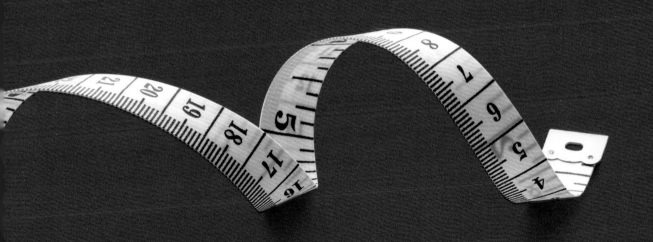

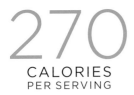

270
CALORIES
PER SERVING

lemon and parmesan chicken

SERVES 4

PREP: 5 MINUTES

COOK: 25 MINUTES

40g fresh white
breadcrumbs
finely grated zest of
½ lemon
15g Parmesan cheese,
finely grated
oil, for spraying or brushing
4 boneless, skinless chicken
breasts (each about 175g)
50g light soft cheese with
garlic and herbs
2 rashers smoked back
bacon (about 65g)
ground black pepper
everyday salad (see right),
to serve

This crunchy chicken has a hidden layer of lower-calorie garlic and herb cheese that helps keep it deliciously moist. I like to serve it simply with everyday salad (see below) but you could add a few new potatoes if you like. This is one occasion where fresh breadcrumbs work much better than dried.

Preheat the oven to 220°C/Fan 200°C/Gas 7. Mix the breadcrumbs, lemon zest and Parmesan together. Spray or brush a shallow ovenproof dish or baking tray with oil. Place the chicken breasts in the dish and spread evenly with cheese.

Press the breadcrumbs on top of the chicken and season with freshly ground black pepper.

Cut any visible fat off the bacon and slice into strips. Scatter over the chicken.

Bake for 25 minutes or until the topping is crisp and lightly browned and the chicken is cooked through.

Everyday salad: Toss the leaves from 2 baby gem lettuces with half a sliced cucumber, a 50g bag spinach, watercress and rocket salad, 200g halved cherry tomatoes and 4 sliced spring onions. Drizzle with 2 teaspoons balsamic vinegar whisked with 1 tablespoon extra virgin olive oil.
Serves 4. Calories per serving: 53

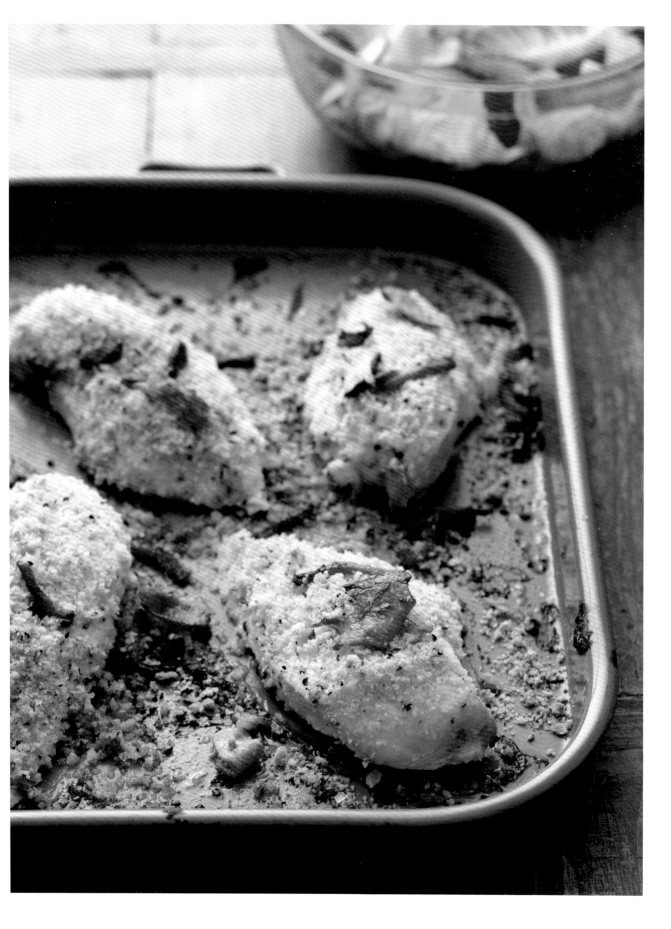

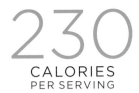

230
CALORIES
PER SERVING

lemon chicken

SERVES 4

PREP: 15 MINUTES

COOK: 15 MINUTES

3 boneless, skinless
chicken breasts

1 tbsp sunflower oil

2 mixed colour peppers,
deseeded and cut into
2.5cm chunks

2 medium carrots, peeled
and thinly sliced

200g long-stemmed
broccoli, cut in half
lengthways if thick

finely grated zest of 1 lemon

2 large garlic cloves,
very thinly sliced

1 tbsp cornflour

2 tbsp dark soy sauce

3 tbsp fresh lemon juice

300ml chicken stock
(made with ½ chicken
stock cube)

8 spring onions, trimmed
and cut into roughly
2cm lengths

This zingy stir-fry is very filling and packed with colourful vegetables. Serve with small portions of rice to soak up the tangy lemon sauce.

Cut the chicken breasts into roughly 2.5cm chunks. Heat 1 teaspoon of the oil in a large, deep non-stick frying pan or wok over a high heat and stir-fry the chicken for 3 minutes, or until lightly browned. Tip the chicken into a clean bowl.

Heat the rest of the oil in the pan and stir-fry the peppers and carrots for 3 minutes. Add the broccoli, lemon zest and garlic and cook for 2 minutes more.

Mix the cornflour with the soy sauce and lemon juice in a small bowl. Pour the stock into the pan with the vegetables and add the chicken. Stir in the lemon juice mixture and the spring onions.

Bring to a simmer and cook for 2–3 minutes more or until the chicken is cooked through and the sauce has thickened, stirring regularly.

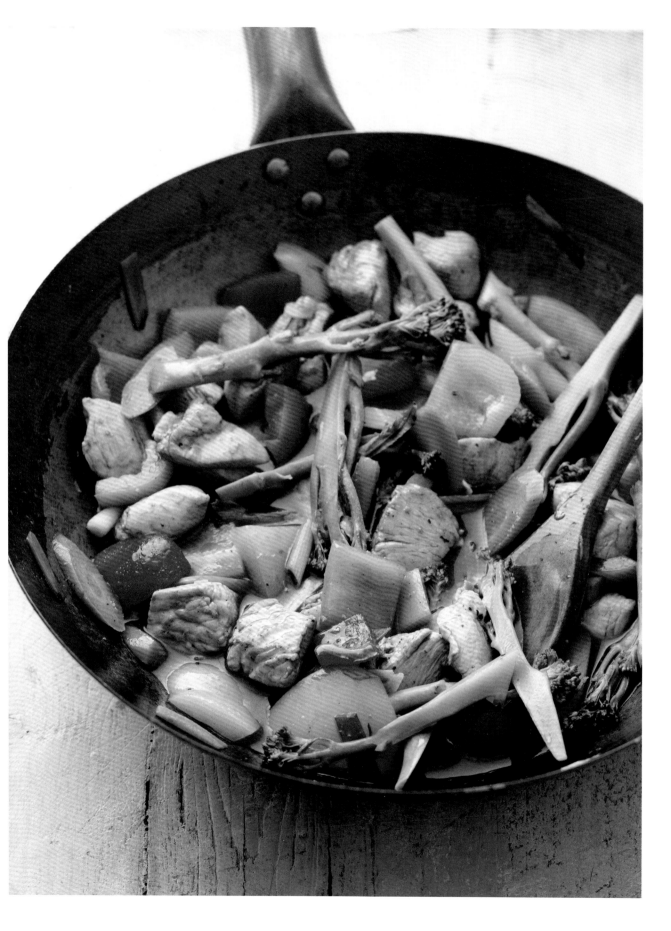

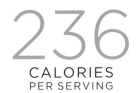

chicken with saffron, pistachios and honey

SERVES 4
PREP: 10 MINUTES
COOK: 25 MINUTES

150ml hot chicken stock
   (made with ½ chicken
   stock cube)
good pinch saffron
1 tbsp harissa paste,
   from a jar
finely grated zest of
   ½ lemon
4 boneless, skinless chicken
   breasts (each about 175g)
2 tsp ras-el-hanout
2 tbsp clear honey
15g shelled pistachio nuts
ground black pepper
orange and coriander
   couscous (see right),
   to serve

Part roasting and part braising ensures that these Moroccan-style chicken breasts remain tender and come with their own fragrant sauce – just right for couscous or rice to soak up. Try serving with my orange and coriander couscous (see below) and lightly dressed salad.

Preheat the oven to 220°C/Fan 200°C/Gas 7. In a large jug, mix together the stock, saffron, harissa and lemon zest. Pour the mixture into a roasting tin or shallow ovenproof dish big enough to hold four chicken breasts fairly snugly.

Slash each chicken breast 3-4 times then season all over with the ras-el-hanout and place them in the stock mixture. The liquid should rise around 1cm up the sides of each breast.

Drizzle over the honey and season with black pepper. Roughly chop the pistachio nuts and sprinkle on top.

Bake for 25 minutes or until the chicken is lightly browned and cooked through. Divide the chicken between four warmed plates and spoon over the fragrant sauce.

Orange and coriander couscous: Put 125g couscous in a heatproof bowl and toss with the finely grated zest of ½ orange. Stir in 200ml hot chicken stock, made with ½ chicken stock cube. Cover and leave to stand for 5 minutes. Uncover and stir in 3 heaped tablespoons roughly chopped coriander and a good grind of black pepper. Serves 4. Calories per serving: 118

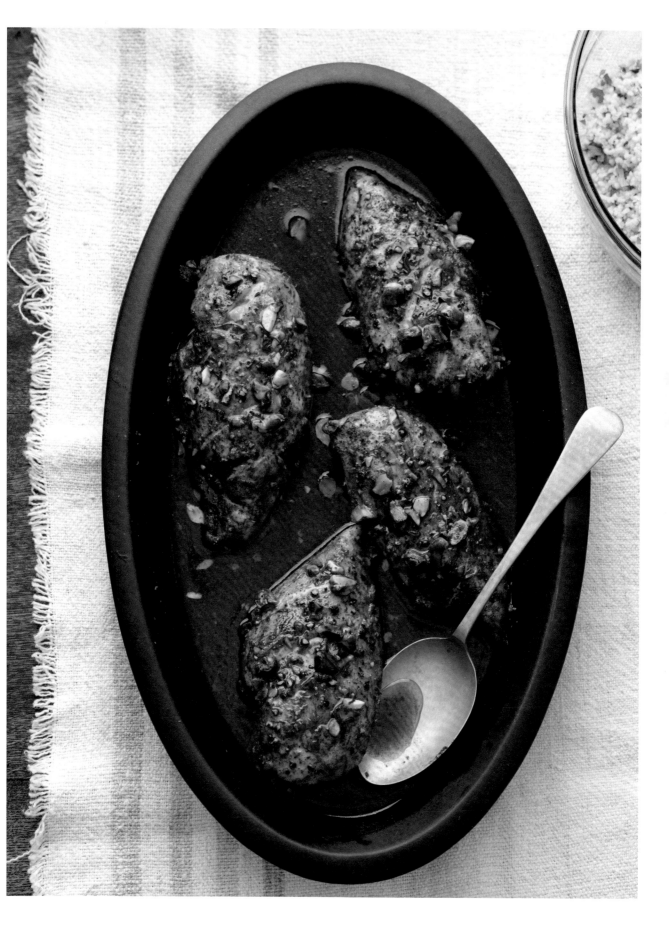

323
CALORIES
PER SERVING

turkey chilli

SERVES 4

PREP: 10 MINUTES

COOK: 15 MINUTES

1 tbsp sunflower oil
500g minced turkey breast
1 large onion,
    finely chopped
2 garlic cloves, finely
    chopped
1–2 tsp hot chilli powder,
    depending on taste
2 tsp smoked paprika,
    (not hot smoked)
2 tsp ground cumin
2 tsp ground coriander
2 tbsp plain flour
200ml chicken stock (made
    with 1 chicken stock cube)
400g can chopped
    tomatoes
1 tsp dried oregano
400g can red kidney beans,
    drained and rinsed
flaked sea salt
freshly ground black pepper

TO SERVE
100ml soured cream
freshly chopped coriander,
    to garnish (optional)

Flat freeze the cooled
chilli in zip-seal bags for
up to 3 months. Reheat
from frozen with an extra
splash of water in a large,
wide-based saucepan over
a medium heat until piping
hot throughout, stirring
regularly.

A lower-fat alternative to beef chilli and much cheaper too.
Make sure you buy minced turkey or chicken breast as the
dark meat will add extra calories. Serve with freshly cooked
vegetables or a small portion of rice and a big salad.

Heat the oil in a large, deep non-stick frying pan or wok and
fry the turkey and onion for 5 minutes until coloured all over,
squishing the mince against the side of the pan to break up
the meat. Season with salt and pepper.

Stir in the garlic, chilli and spices and cook for 2–3 minutes
more, while stirring. Sprinkle over the flour and stir well.
Gradually stir in the stock and then add the tomatoes,
oregano and beans.

Bring to a gentle simmer, stirring continuously for 5 minutes or
until the turkey is tender and the sauce is thick. Serve topped
with spoonfuls of soured cream and chopped coriander, if using.

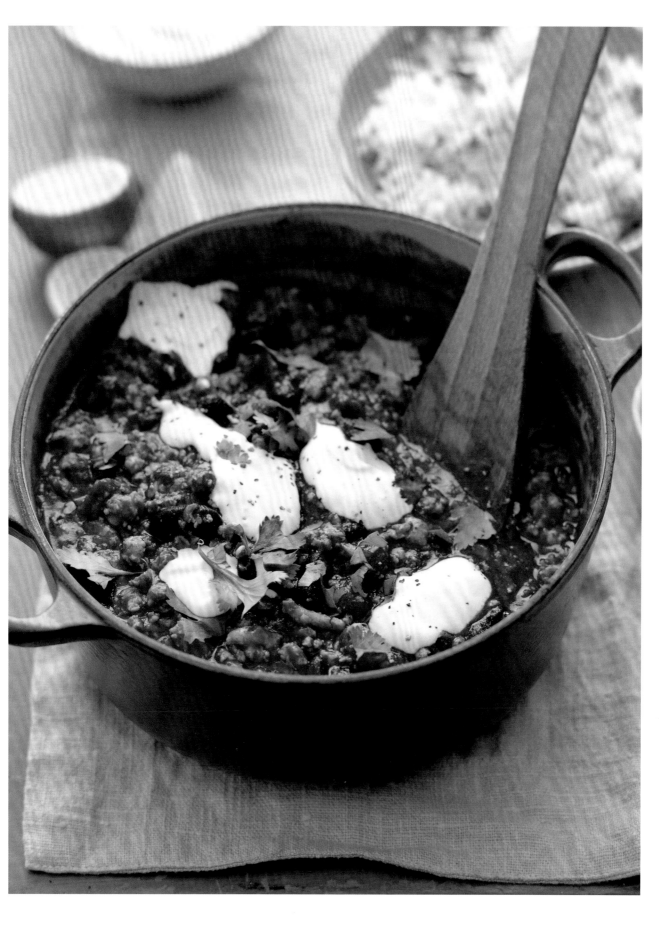

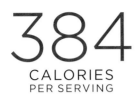

384
CALORIES
PER SERVING

mediterranean
turkey burgers

SERVES 4

PREP: 15 MINUTES

COOK: 20 MINUTES

1 medium-large courgette
(about 250g)
500g minced turkey breast
4 spring onions, trimmed
and very thinly sliced
2 tbsp sun-dried tomato
pesto
finely grated zest of 1 lemon
½ tsp flaked sea salt
oil, for spraying or brushing
2 ciabatta rolls (each
about 100g)
1–2 large ripe tomatoes,
sliced
handful of fresh basil leaves
125g ball light mozzarella,
drained and sliced
ground black pepper

Grated courgette keeps these burgers moist, and sun-dried tomato pesto adds sweetness and flavour. Half of a ciabatta roll should be plenty for one serving, so don't be tempted to eat more. If you don't fancy a roll, you can serve with a small portion of 5% or less fat oven chips instead.

Preheat the oven to 220°C/Fan 200°C/Gas 7. Finely grate the courgette then squeeze the excess water from it with your hands over the sink.

Put the courgette in a large bowl and add the minced turkey, spring onions, tomato pesto, lemon zest, salt and ground black pepper. Combine with your hands until thoroughly mixed. Form the mince mixture into four balls and flatten into burger shapes.

Brush or spray a little oil over a baking tray. Place the burgers on the tray and brush with more oil. Bake for 10 minutes, then turn over and bake for a further 8 minutes, or until lightly browned and cooked through.

While the burgers are cooking, cut the ciabatta rolls in half and toast or griddle until nicely browned. Place the hot burgers on top of the halved rolls with sliced tomatoes, basil leaves and mozzarella. Serve with a colourful salad.

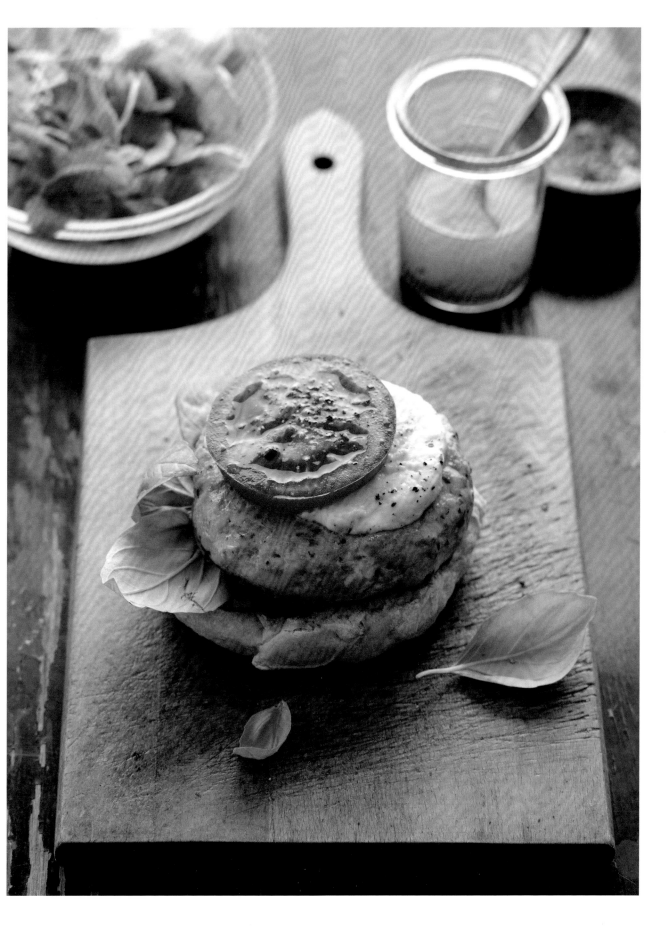

293
CALORIES
PER SERVING

breton chicken

SERVES 2
PREP: 10 MINUTES
COOK: 25–30 MINUTES

1 garlic clove, crushed
15g flat leaf parsley, leaves
    finely chopped
1 tbsp mild olive oil
    or sunflower oil
2 boneless, skinless chicken
    breasts (each about 175g)
1 medium leek, trimmed
    and cut into roughly
    1cm slices
1 tsp cornflour
2 tbsp white wine
2 tbsp half fat crème fraiche
5 tbsp cold water
flaked sea salt
ground black pepper

These tender baked chicken breasts are cooked on a bed of leeks and served with a simple, creamy white wine sauce that cooks and thickens in the same pan as the chicken. I like to boil a few runner beans and carrots or a portion of peas to serve alongside.

Preheat the oven to 220°C/Fan 200°C/Gas 7. Mix the garlic, parsley and 2 teaspoons of the oil in a small bowl. Slash each chicken breast 3–4 times then rub the herb mixture all over, especially into the cuts.

Spread the sliced leek loosely over the base of a small roasting or ovenproof dish – the chicken breasts need to fit fairly snugly, so it shouldn't be larger than 16 x 20cm. Toss lightly in the remaining teaspoon of oil. Place the chicken breasts on top, season with salt and pepper and bake for 15 minutes.

While the chicken is baking, mix the cornflour and wine in a bowl until smooth and whisk in the crème fraiche and water. Take the chicken breasts out of the oven and pour the sauce over them. Return to the oven for a further 10-15 minutes or until the chicken is cooked through.

Transfer the chicken to two warmed plates. Stir the leeks and cream sauce together well and spoon over the top.

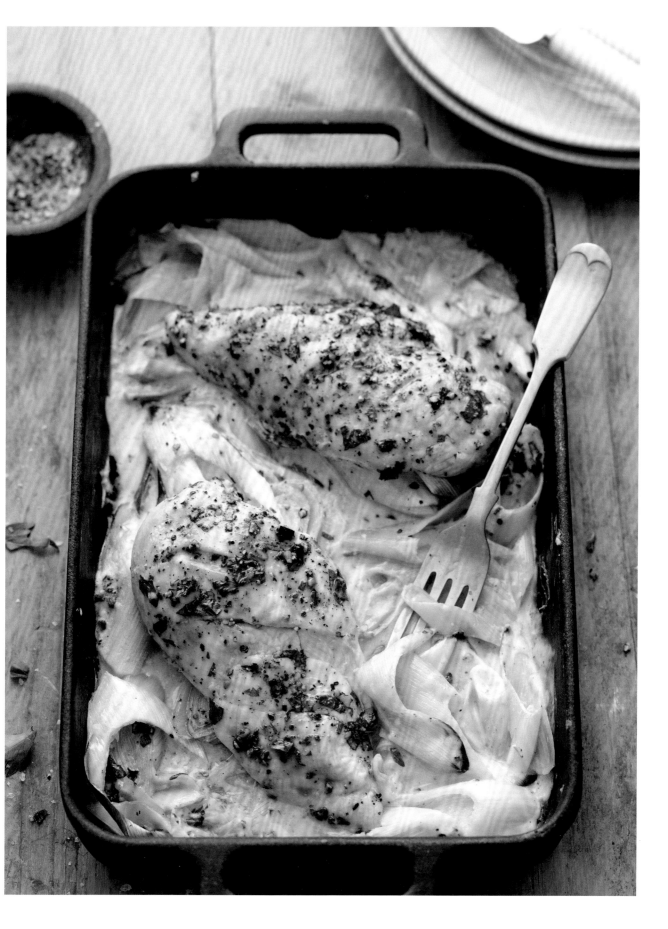

282 CALORIES PER SERVING

super-quick coq au vin

SERVES 4
PREP: 15 MINUTES
COOK: 35 MINUTES

16 shallots
8 boneless, skinless chicken thighs (about 750g)
1 tbsp mild olive oil
4 rashers smoked back bacon (about 125g)
150g baby button mushrooms, halved if large
100ml Marsala or Madeira wine
150ml chicken stock (made with ½ chicken stock cube)
flaked sea salt
ground black pepper

A deliciously rich supper dish that's very simple to prepare. Peeling the shallots takes a little time but the rest can be knocked together easily. Serve with small portions of mashed potato or white bean mash (see page 80), green beans and carrots.

Preheat the oven to 200°C/Fan 180°C/Gas 6. Place the shallots in a large heatproof bowl and cover with just-boiled water. Leave to stand for 5 minutes to allow the skins to loosen. Drain the shallots in a colander and rinse under cold water.

Using a small knife, cut the base off each shallot and strip off the skin. Don't worry if the shallots split when the skin is lifted – they still count as one shallot. Scatter the shallots over the bottom of a large sturdy roasting tin.

Trim any visible fat off the chicken thighs – a sharp pair of kitchen scissors is good for this. Arrange the thighs in their original shape and place them in the same tin as the shallots. Drizzle with the oil and season all over with salt and ground black pepper. Bake for 20 minutes.

Meanwhile, trim the visible fat off the bacon and cut into 1.5cm slices. Take the roasting tin out of the oven, turn the chicken thighs over and add the bacon and mushrooms. Return to the oven for a further 10–15 minutes or until the chicken is cooked through and lightly browned.

Transfer the contents of the roasting tin to a warmed platter or serving dish. Place the roasting tin on the hob and pour over the Marsala or Madeira and the stock. Bring to a simmer and cook for 2–3 minutes until slightly reduced, stirring to scrape up the juicy bits from the bottom of the pan. Carefully lift the tin and pour the sauce over the chicken.

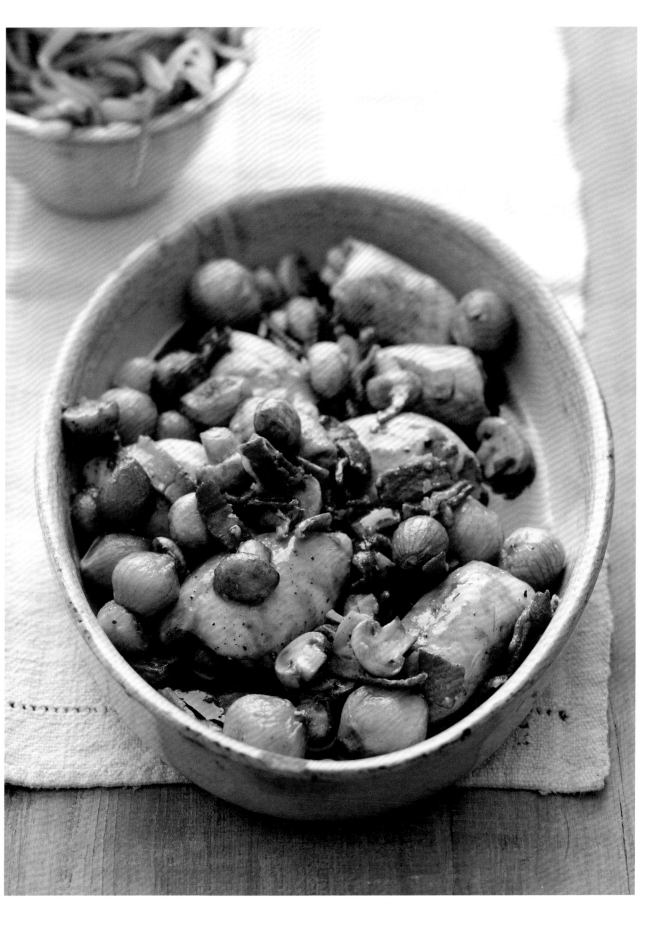

253

CALORIES
PER SERVING

chicken parmigiana

SERVES 6

PREP: 10 MINUTES

COOK: 30 MINUTES

oil, for spraying or brushing
6 boneless, skinless chicken
   breasts (each about 175g)
1 medium onion,
   thinly sliced
2 garlic cloves, crushed
400g can chopped
   tomatoes with herbs
2 tbsp tomato purée
250ml chicken stock (made
   with 1 chicken stock cube)
150ml red wine or
   extra stock
½ tsp dried chilli flakes
   (optional)
50g ready-grated
   mozzarella
flaked sea salt
ground black pepper

Freeze the cooked chicken
and sauce, topped with
uncooked cheese, in
freezer-proof containers
for up to 2 months. Defrost
overnight in the fridge and
reheat in the microwave
until piping hot throughout.
You can also reheat in
a moderate oven for
25–35 minutes.

This is a dish that always goes down well with friends and family – and it freezes brilliantly too. You will need a shallow, wide-based casserole or sauté pan to cook all six breasts at once, but you could make it for four instead and freeze any extra sauce to serve with pasta another time.

Spray or brush a large, deep frying pan, shallow flameproof casserole or sauté pan with oil. Season the chicken breasts on both sides with salt and pepper. Fry the chicken over a medium-high heat for 2 minutes on each side or until nicely browned. Transfer to a plate.

Spray the pan with more oil and add the onion and garlic, reduce the heat and cook for 2–3 minutes, stirring until the onion is lightly coloured. (Do not allow the garlic to burn or it will make the sauce taste bitter.)

Tip the tomatoes into the pan, stir in the tomato purée, chicken stock, wine and chilli flakes, if using. Bring the sauce to a simmer, while stirring.

Place the chicken breasts back in the pan and simmer gently for 18–20 minutes, or until cooked through. Season the sauce with salt and pepper then sprinkle with cheese and simmer for a further 2–3 minutes or until the cheese melts.

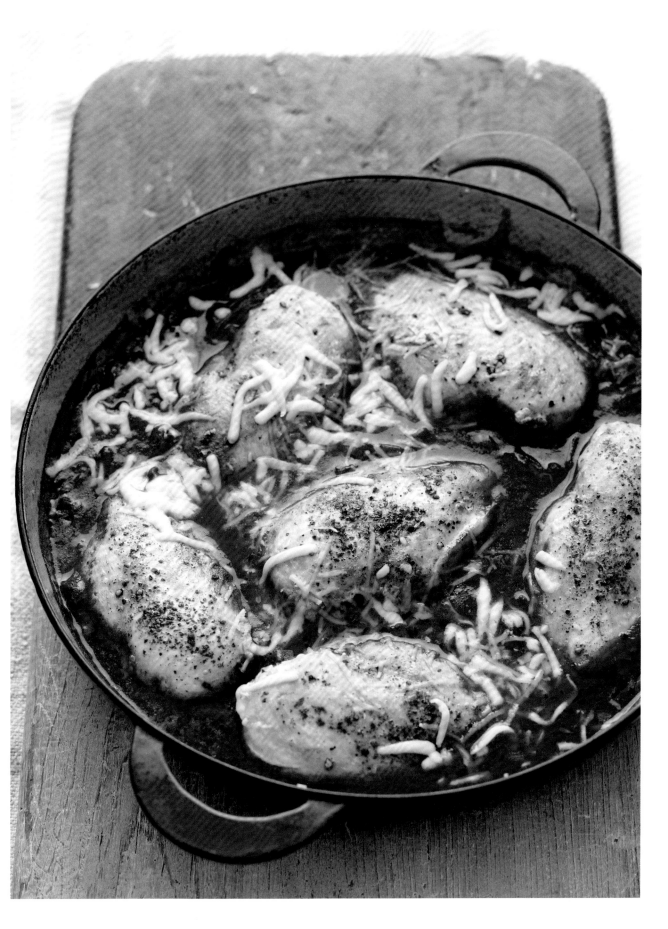

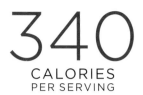

340

CALORIES
PER SERVING

quick chicken curry

SERVES 2
PREP: 10 MINUTES
COOK: 20 MINUTES

2 medium onions, quartered
3 tbsp medium curry
  or balti paste
3 tbsp water
2 boneless, skinless chicken
  breasts
200ml chicken stock
  (made with ½ chicken
  stock cube)
150ml fat-free natural
  yoghurt
20g fresh coriander, leaves
  roughly chopped

Flat freeze the cooled curry
in zip-seal bags for up
to 3 months. Reheat from
frozen with an extra splash
of water in a large, wide-
based saucepan over a
medium heat until piping
hot throughout, stirring
regularly.

A wonderfully creamy curry with very little fat. Using a ready-made paste will save lots of time and it keeps for months in the fridge. Don't use a curry sauce as the results won't be nearly as good. Serve in warm, deep bowls with small portions of rice.

Put the onions and curry paste in a food processor and blitz into a purée. You may need to remove the lid and push the mixture down a couple of times until the right consistency is reached.

Tip the spiced puréed onions into a large, deep non-stick frying pan or wok and cook over a medium heat for 5 minutes, stirring regularly until they begin to soften. Add the water and cook for a further 5 minutes or until the onions are well softened.

Cut the chicken breasts into roughly 3cm chunks and add them to the spiced onions. Increase the heat and cook for 2 minutes, turning regularly.

Pour over the chicken stock and add the yoghurt and coriander. Bring to a gentle simmer. Cook for 8–10 minutes or until the chicken is tender and the sauce is thick, stirring regularly.

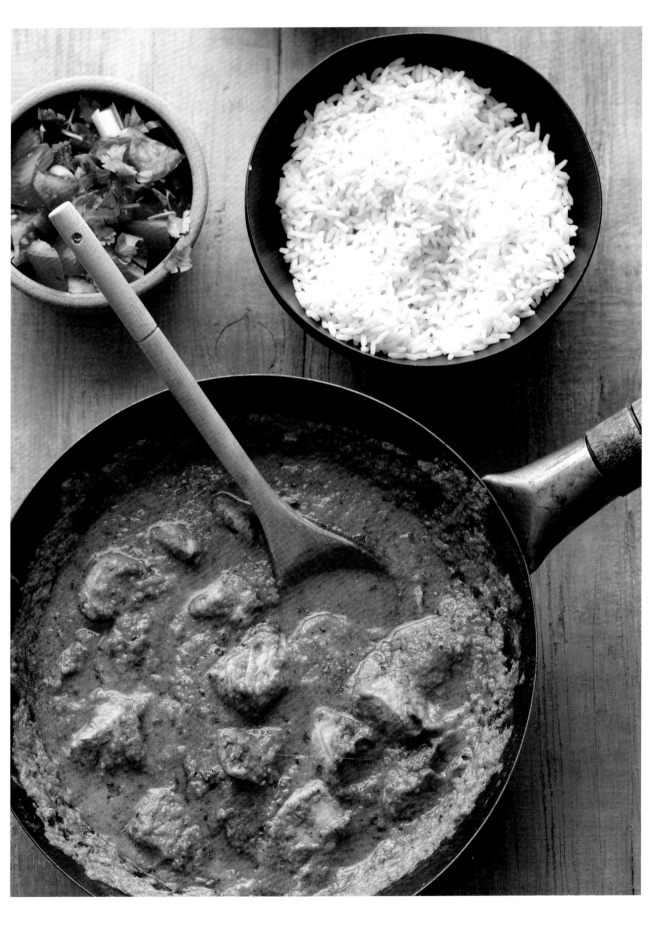

316
CALORIES
PER SERVING

chicken and ham parcels

SERVES 6
PREP: 20 MINUTES
COOK: 20 MINUTES

4 boneless, cooked chicken
  breasts (about 500g),
  skinned
6 spring onions, thinly sliced
4 slices of smoked ham, cut
  into strips (about 120g)
1 tbsp cornflour
200g half-fat crème fraiche
6 filo pastry sheets
  (each about 45g)
oil, for spraying or brushing
ground black pepper

Open freeze the cooled,
unbaked parcels until solid,
then wrap each one tightly
with a double layer of foil.
Put in a freezer bag and
freeze for up to 2 months.
To serve, bake from frozen
as the recipe, increasing the
cooking time by 10 minutes,
until piping hot throughout.

Tip: I've used 45 x 25cm
sheets of filo pastry; if yours
is a different size, you will
need to adjust the folding
method accordingly.

These delicious chicken pies are made with cooked chicken
breasts from the supermarket. You can also use chicken
breasts that you have roasted or poached at home. They're
great served hot or cold and they make an easy addition
to a packed lunch.

Preheat the oven to 200°C/Fan 180°C/Gas 6. Cut or tear the
chicken into roughly 2cm chunks and put the chunks in a bowl.
Add the spring onions, ham and cornflour. Season with black
pepper and toss well together. Add the crème fraiche and
mix well.

Place a sheet of filo pastry on the work surface with the short
end towards you. Spray or brush lightly with the oil. Spoon
a sixth of the chicken mixture into the centre of the bottom
part, leaving a pastry border of 10cm on each long side and
5cm at the bottom.

Fold up the bottom to cover the filling, then fold in the sides
and roll up into a rectangle. Place on a baking sheet and repeat
with the remaining filo and filling. Spray or brush with a little
more oil and sprinkle with a little black pepper.

Bake in the centre of the oven for about 20 minutes or until
the pastry is golden brown and the filling is hot and bubbling.

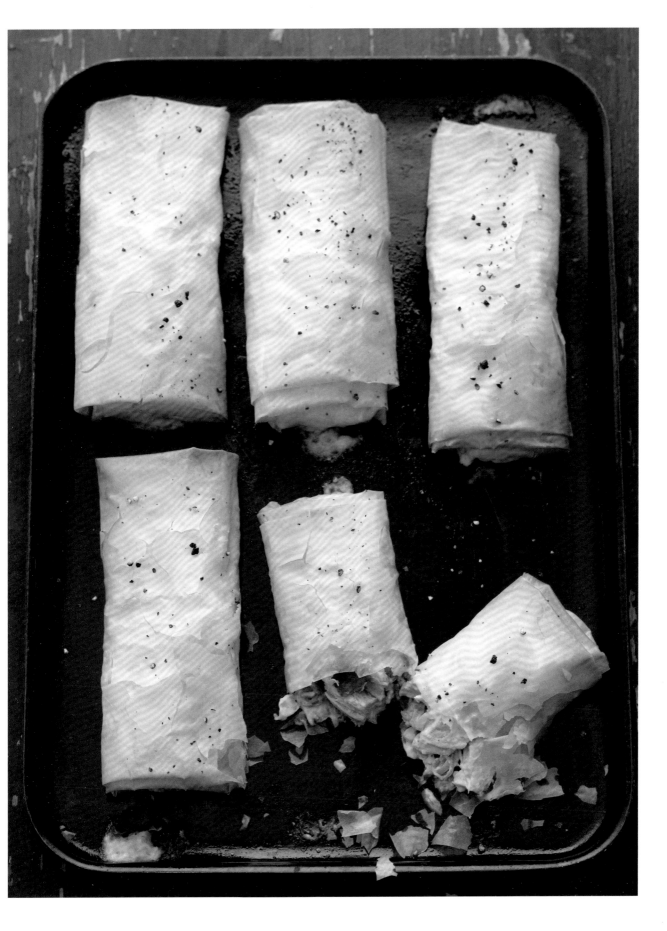

158

CALORIES
PER SERVING

turkey lettuce wraps

SERVES 4
PREP: 5 MINUTES
COOK: 10 MINUTES

oil, for spraying or brushing
500g turkey or chicken
    breast mince
15g chunk fresh root ginger,
    peeled and finely grated
8 spring onions, trimmed
    and thinly sliced
1 long red chilli, thinly sliced
    (deseed first if you like)
1 tbsp dark soy sauce
1 tbsp Thai fish sauce
    (nam pla)
1 iceberg lettuce, leaves
    separated (or 3 little
    gem lettuces)
lime wedges, for squeezing

These are great fun for a casual dinner – you can put the turkey mixture in the middle of the table and everyone can just help themselves.

Spray or brush a large non-stick frying pan or wok with the oil and place over a high heat. Add the turkey or chicken mince and cook for 3 minutes, using two wooden spoons to break up the meat as it cooks.

Stir the ginger, spring onions and chilli into the pan and fry the mince for a further minute or until the turkey or chicken is cooked – it should be completely white with no pink remaining. Add the soy sauce and fish sauce and toss them through the mince. Tip everything into a bowl.

To serve, scoop the hot mince mixture into the lettuce leaves, squeeze over a little lime juice and eat with your fingers.

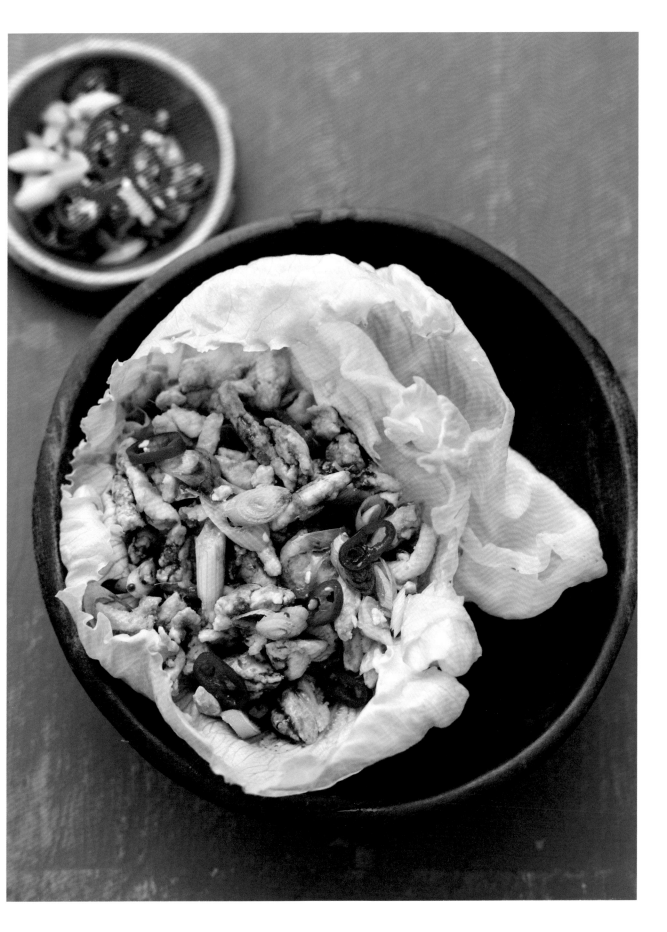

256
CALORIES
PER SERVING

cheat's chicken casserole

SERVES 6
PREP: 10 MINUTES
COOK: 1 HOUR

12 boneless, skinless chicken
   thighs (about 1kg)
3 smoked back bacon
   rashers (about 90g)
oil, for spraying or brushing
1 medium onion,
   thinly sliced
500g frozen casserole
   vegetables
400g can chopped
   tomatoes with herbs
1 chicken stock cube
150ml white wine or
   extra water
2 tbsp tomato purée
flaked sea salt
ground black pepper

Freeze the cooled chicken
casserole in freezer-proof
containers for up to
3 months. Defrost overnight
in the fridge and heat
through in a large wide-
based saucepan over a
medium heat until piping
hot throughout, stirring
occasionally.

You can find frozen casserole vegetables – a combination of prepared carrots, swedes, turnips, celery and button onions – in the freezer aisle of most large supermarkets and they make a great standby for dishes like this. Serve just as it is or with a small portion of rice or mashed potatoes to soak up the rich, tomato sauce, and some peas.

Trim any visible fat from the chicken thighs – a pair of kitchen scissors is good for this. Cut each thigh in half and season all over with salt and pepper. Trim any visible fat off the bacon and cut into 2cm strips.

Preheat the oven to 200°C/Fan 180°C/Gas 6. Brush or spray a large flameproof casserole with oil and place over a medium-high heat. Fry the onion and bacon for 5 minutes or until the onion starts to soften, stirring regularly.

Add the chicken and cook for 4–5 minutes, turning every now and then until sealed on all sides. Tip the vegetables into the pan, add the tomatoes and crumble over the stock cube.

Fill the tomato can with water and pour it into the dish. Add the wine and tomato purée and bring to the boil. Cover with a lid and cook in the oven for 45 minutes or until the chicken and vegetables are tender.

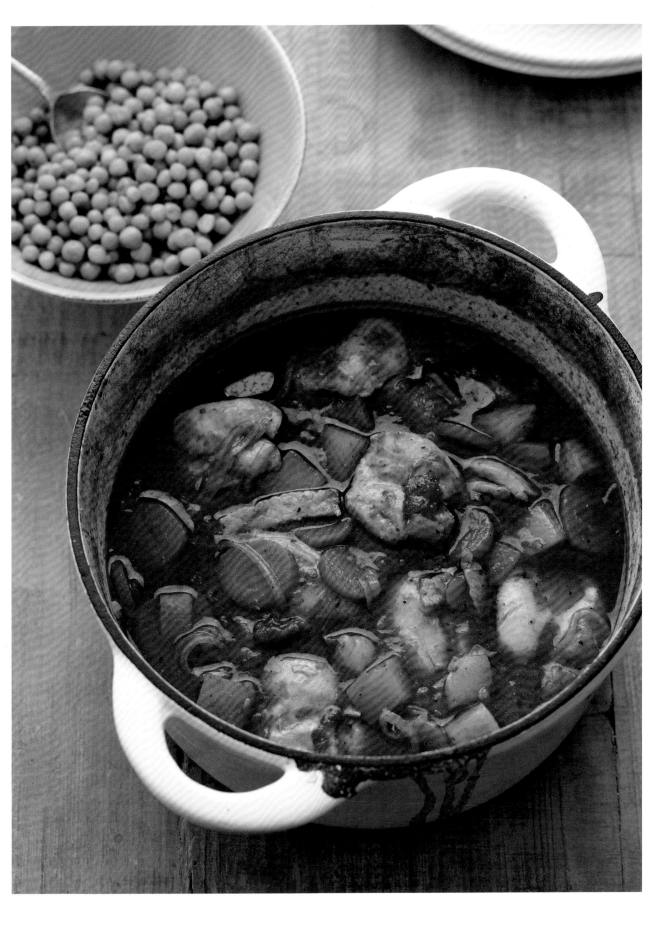

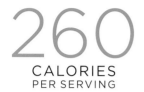

martini chicken

SERVES 4

PREP TIME: 10 MINUTES

COOK: 25 MINUTES

4 boneless, skinless chicken
breasts (each about 175g)
4 slices of Parma ham
or prosciutto
8 fresh sage leaves
oil, for spraying or brushing
300ml chicken stock
(made with ½ chicken
stock cube)
100ml Martini Rosso
flaked sea salt
ground black pepper
lemon and parsley carrots
(see right), to serve

I love the rich flavour and colour that sweet Martini brings
to this dish. It really complements the saltiness of the ham;
but you could use Marsala or Madeira instead. Pan-frying the
chicken breasts and then simmering them in the stock helps
them remain succulent. Serve with carrots (see below) and
boiled or mashed potatoes if you like.

Season the chicken breasts on both sides with salt and pepper
and wrap each breast with a slice of Parma ham or prosciutto,
tucking a couple of sage leaves under each piece.

Spray or brush a deep non-stick frying pan or sauté pan with
oil. Fry the chicken over a medium-high heat for 3 minutes
on each side or until nicely browned.

Add the chicken stock and Martini to the pan and bring
to the boil. Reduce the heat and simmer gently for 15–20
minutes, turning the chicken occasionally until tender
and cooked through.

Transfer the chicken to warmed plates and increase the heat
under the pan. Boil the sauce for 1–2 minutes, stirring constantly
until well reduced and thick enough to lightly coat the back
of the spoon. Pour the sauce over the chicken and serve.

Lemon and parsley carrots: Boil 500g peeled or scrubbed
and halved Chantenay carrots for 10–12 minutes or until tender.
Drain and return to the pan. Add a 15g knob of butter, the
finely grated zest of ½ lemon, 2 tablespoons finely chopped
parsley, a good pinch of salt and lots of ground black pepper.
Toss over a low heat for 1–2 minutes until the parsley softens
and the butter melts and lightly glazes the carrots. Serves 4.
Calories per serving: 66

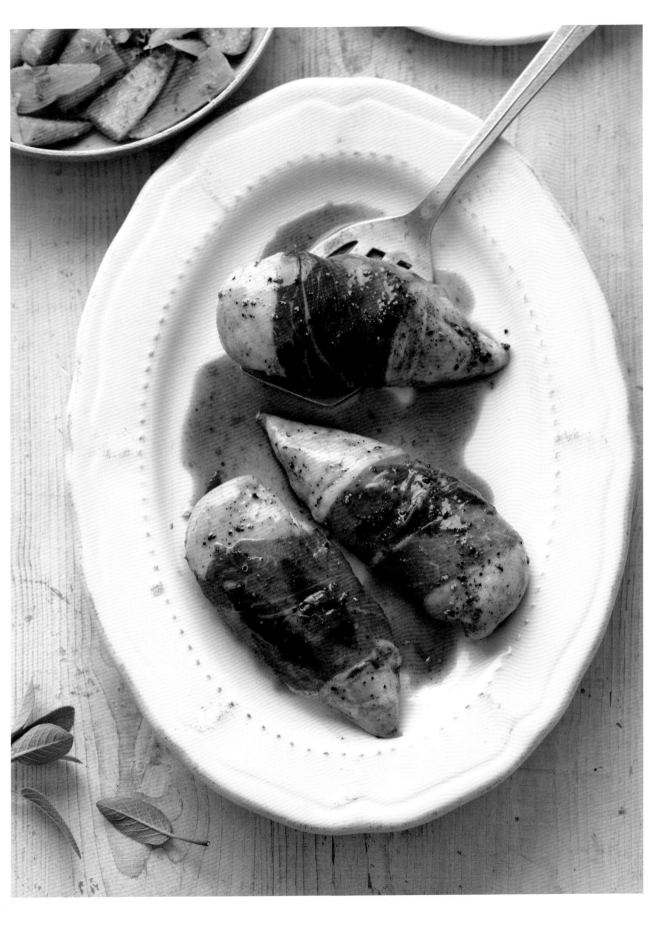

181
CALORIES
PER SERVING

turkey bolognese with cheat's spaghetti

SERVES 6
PREP: 15 MINUTES
COOK: 30–35 MINUTES

1 tbsp sunflower oil
500g minced turkey breast
1 medium onion,
    finely chopped
2 celery sticks, thinly sliced
2 medium carrots, peeled
    and finely diced
2 garlic cloves, crushed
250g baby button
    mushrooms, halved
2 tbsp plain flour
125ml red wine or water
2 x 400g cans chopped
    tomatoes with herbs
2 tbsp tomato purée
200ml chicken stock
    (made with 1 chicken
    stock cube)
2 bay leaves
flaked sea salt
ground black pepper
cheat's spaghetti
    (see right)
fresh basil, to garnish
    (optional)

Flat freeze the cooled
Bolognese in zip-seal bags
for up to 3 months. Reheat
from frozen with an extra
splash of water in a large,
wide-based saucepan over
a medium heat until piping
hot throughout, stirring
regularly.

Using minced turkey instead of beef cuts the cooking time
and reduces the fat content of this Bolognese sauce. Cheat's
spaghetti is one of my favourites and something I go back
to time and time again. It's important to use a pale white
cabbage so it really does resemble pasta. An average serving
of spaghetti contains around 220 calories – a serving of
cabbage 'spaghetti' has 68 calories.

Heat the oil in a large, deep non-stick saucepan or sauté pan.
Fry the mince with the onion, celery, carrots and garlic in the
pan over a medium heat for 5 minutes. Squash the meat with
a wooden spoon to break up any large lumps.

Add the mushrooms and fry with the mince and vegetables
for a further 2–3 minutes. Stir in the flour then the wine or
water, tomatoes, tomato purée and stock. Add the bay leaves,
season with ground black pepper, give it a good stir
and bring to a gentle simmer.

Simmer gently for 20–25 minutes, stirring occasionally, until
the turkey and vegetables are tender and the sauce is thick.
Add salt and pepper to taste. Serve with the freshly boiled
cabbage 'spaghetti' or small portions of pasta and a big
salad. Garnish with fresh basil if you like.

Cheat's spaghetti: Cut 1 medium white cabbage (around
1.2kg) in half and remove the core. Very thinly slice the cabbage
and then rub it through your fingers to separate the strands.
Put the cabbage into a large saucepan and add enough just-
boiled water to rise 5cm up the sides. Cover with a lid and boil
for 4–5 minutes or until tender, stirring twice. Drain well.
Serves 4. Calories per serving: 68

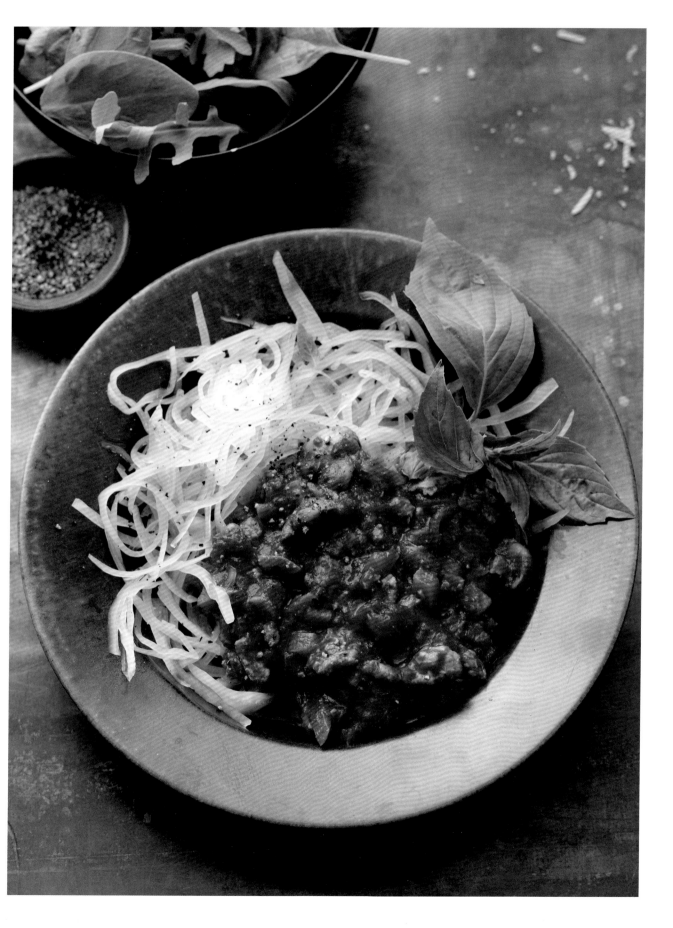

275

CALORIES
PER SERVING

tex mex chicken tart

SERVES 4

PREP: 10 MINUTES

COOK: 25 MINUTES

oil, for spraying or brushing
2 small courgettes (each
    about 150g), trimmed and
    cut into 1.5cm slices
2 mixed colour peppers,
    deseeded and cut into
    roughly 2cm chunks
1 medium red onion,
    cut into 12 wedges
4 sheets filo pastry
    (each about 45g)
200g pot fresh tomato
    salsa sauce
1 cooked chicken breast
    (about 125g), skinned
50g ready-grated
    mozzarella

This colourful tart makes a simple lunch served with a big,
lightly dressed salad. You can make it veggie-friendly by
leaving out the chicken too. Filo pastry is very easy to use
as a tart base and contains far fewer calories than puff
pastry, even when lightly brushed or sprayed with oil.

Preheat the oven to 220°C/Fan 200°C/Gas 7. Brush or spray
a large non-stick frying pan or wok with oil. Add the vegetables
to the pan and stir-fry for 5 minutes or until nicely coloured.
Tip into a large bowl.

Line a large baking tray with baking parchment and place
one of the pastry sheets on top. Spray or brush lightly with oil
and top with a second sheet. Spray or brush with more oil
and repeat the layers twice more. Spread roughly with
the salsa sauce.

Tear the chicken breast into strips and scatter over the
salsa. Arrange the cooked vegetables on top. Sprinkle with
the mozzarella. Bake for 15–20 minutes or until the pastry
is golden brown and crisp.

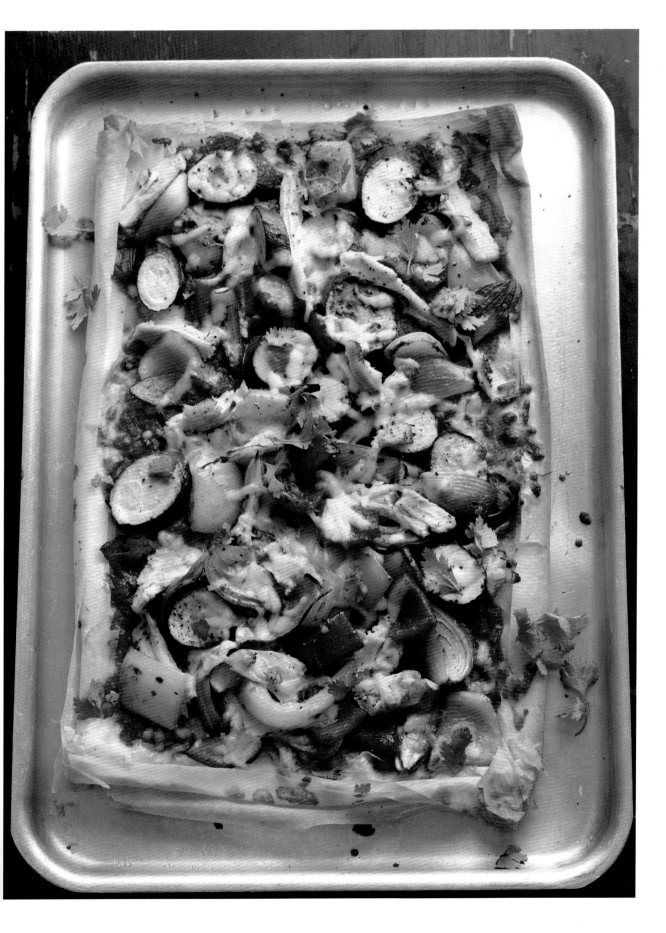

257
CALORIES
PER SERVING

tom's paprika chicken

SERVES 6

PREP: 15 MINUTES

COOK: 50 MINUTES

1 tbsp sunflower oil
2 medium onions,
   thinly sliced
12 boneless, skinless chicken
   thighs (about 1kg)
2 garlic cloves, crushed
1 tbsp paprika (not smoked)
1–2 tsp hot smoked paprika,
   depending on taste
400g can chopped
   tomatoes with herbs
300ml chicken stock (made
   with 1 chicken stock cube)
100ml white wine or
   extra stock
3 mixed colour peppers,
   deseeded and cut into
   roughly 4cm chunks
flaked sea salt
ground black pepper
soured cream, to serve

Freeze in freezer-proof
containers for up to
4 months. Defrost overnight
in the fridge and reheat in a
large saucepan or casserole,
stirring occasionally until
piping hot throughout.

Tip: I love Tom's paprika
chicken topped with
spoonfuls of soured cream
but you could also use
yoghurt or leave it plain.
Soured cream contains
31 calories per tablespoon
and fat-free yoghurt
contains 8 calories.

I was introduced to this dish by a Hungarian friend named
Tom, who is an excellent cook. My version has fewer calories
but is full of paprika and has a lovely rich colour. Serve with
rice, noodles or mashed potatoes, topped with spoonfuls
of soured cream.

Heat the oil in a large, wide-based non-stick saucepan or
flameproof casserole and fry the onions over a medium-high
heat for 3 minutes until lightly coloured, stirring regularly.

Trim any visible fat from the chicken and cut the thighs
in half. Season the chicken all over with salt and ground
black pepper and add to the pan.

Fry for 5 minutes or until sealed on all sides. Stir in the garlic
and both paprikas and cook for a few seconds, stirring
continuously. Tip the tomatoes into the pan and pour over the
chicken stock and wine.

Bring to a gentle simmer, then cover the pan loosely with
a lid and cook for 20 minutes, stirring occasionally.

Add the peppers to the chicken and simmer without covering
for a further 15 minutes, stirring regularly until the sauce is
thick and the chicken is tender. Garnish with roughly chopped
parsley if you like.

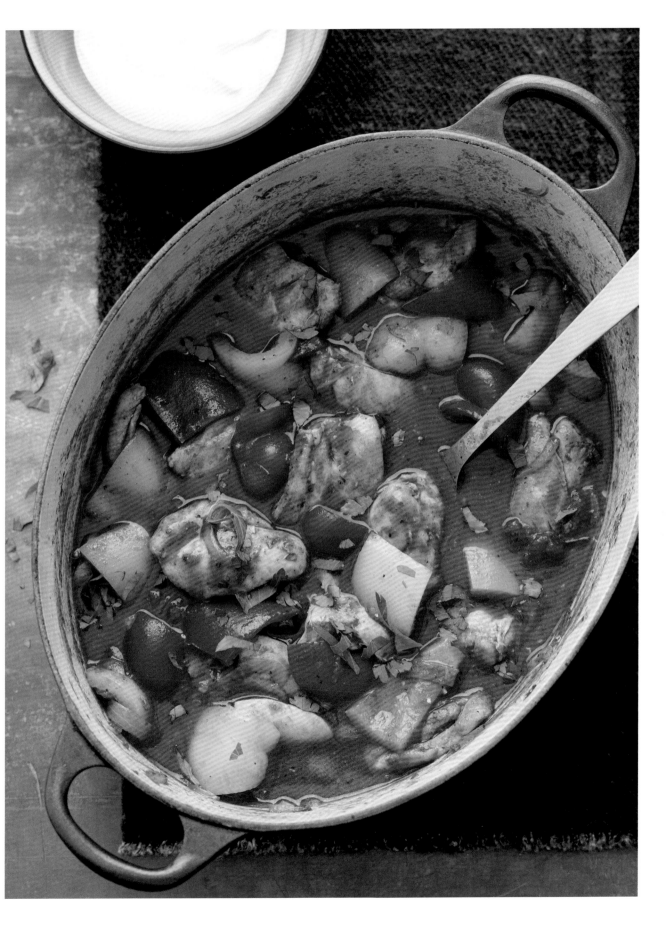

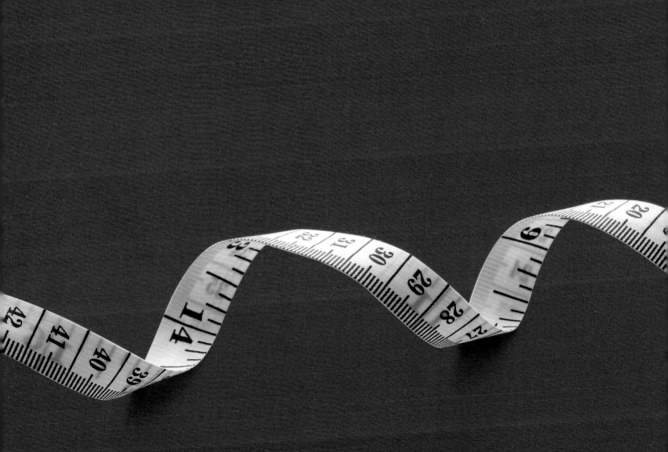

pork, lamb and beef

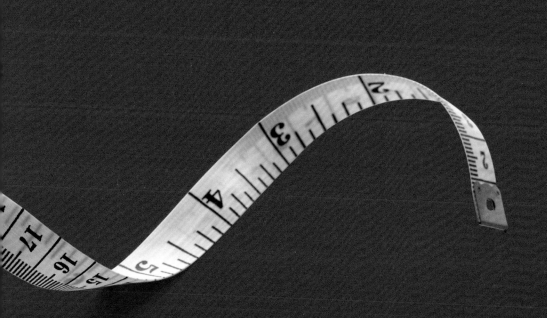

256

spaghetti on fire

4 rashers of smoked back
   bacon (about 125g)
oil, for spraying or brushing
1 medium onion,
   thinly sliced
2 mixed colour peppers,
   deseeded and cut into
   roughly 2cm chunks
2 medium courgettes, cut
   into roughly 2cm chunks
2 garlic cloves, thinly sliced
1–2 tsp dried chilli flakes,
   depending on taste
2 x 400g cans chopped
   tomatoes with herbs
175g dried spaghetti
ground black pepper
grated Parmesan cheese
   (optional)
fresh torn basil leaves,
   to garnish (optional)

Flat freeze the cooled pasta
and sauce in zip-seal bags.
Defrost overnight in the
fridge and reheat in the
microwave or in a saucepan
over a medium heat, stirring
regularly until piping hot.

A fiery pasta dish based on spaghetti Amatriciana, but with a little less pasta and lots of extra vegetables. Sprinkle each portion with a tablespoon of freshly grated Parmesan and add an extra 21 calories per serving.

Trim all visible fat off the bacon with a good pair of kitchen scissors. Cut the bacon into roughly 2cm strips. Spray or brush a large non-stick sauté pan or deep frying pan with oil and fry the bacon over a medium heat for 2 minutes or until lightly browned. Tip onto a plate and set aside.

Spray or brush the pan with a little more oil and cook the onion for 2 minutes or until beginning to soften, stirring regularly. Add the peppers and courgettes and cook over a medium-high heat for 5 minutes until lightly browned.

Add the garlic and chilli flakes and cook for a few seconds more, while stirring. Tip the tomatoes into the pan, return the bacon and bring to a gentle simmer over a low heat. Cook for 15 minutes, stirring regularly.

While the sauce is cooking, half fill a large pan with water and bring to the boil. Add the pasta and return to the boil. Cook for 10–12 minutes or until just tender, stirring occasionally.

Drain the pasta in a colander and return to the pan. Stir in the tomato sauce and toss until combined. Season with ground black pepper. Divide between warmed bowls and sprinkle with grated Parmesan, if using, and fresh basil leaves if you like. Serve with the everyday salad (see page 30) or any colourful mixed salad.

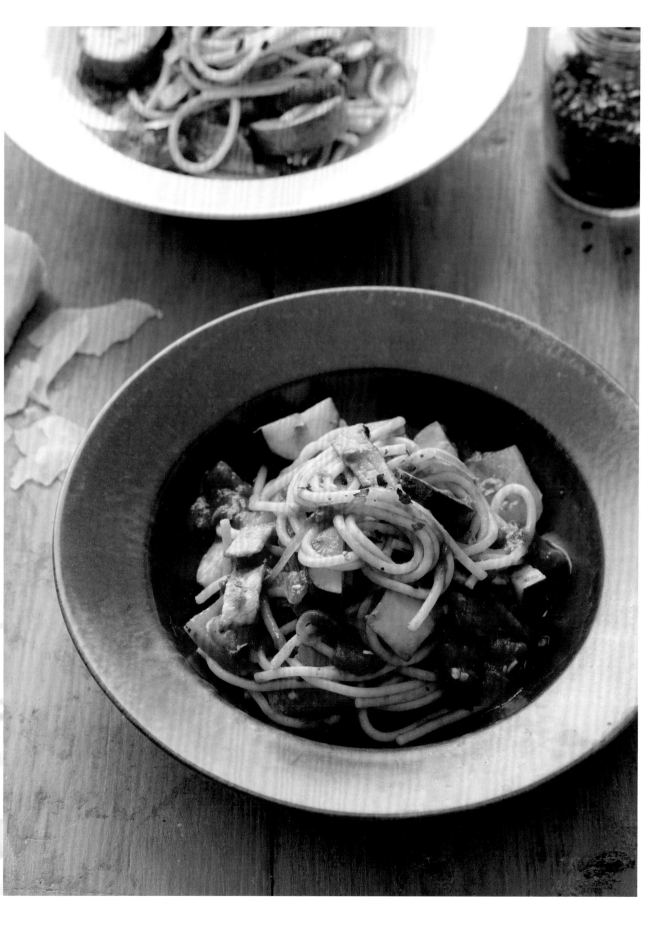

516
CALORIES
PER SERVING

sirloin steak, chips and béarnaise sauce

SERVES 4

PREP: 10 MINUTES

COOK: 20 MINUTES

400g straight cut oven
   chips (5% or less fat)
4 x 200g sirloin steaks
2 tsp coarsely ground
   black pepper
oil, for brushing or spraying
flaked sea salt

FOR THE MOCK
BÉARNAISE SAUCE
4 tbsp white wine vinegar
1 small bay leaf
4 peppercorns
½ tsp flaked sea salt,
   plus extra to taste
200ml semi-skimmed milk
15g cornflour
20g butter
1 tbsp finely chopped
   fresh tarragon
3 large egg yolks
ground black pepper

Note: This recipe contains
lightly cooked eggs.

Lean steak makes a delicious and filling meal. When
you are short of time, frozen oven chips make a simple
accompaniment. Look for the ones containing 5% or less
fat per 100g and you can still enjoy a small portion and
stay within your calorie allowance. My mock Béarnaise
sauce contains 20g butter rather than 200g – a huge
saving in calories.

Preheat the oven to 220°C/Fan 200°C/Gas 7. Scatter the
chips over a baking tray and cook in the oven for 18–20 minutes
or according to the pack instructions until hot and crisp.

Meanwhile, make the mock Béarnaise. Put the vinegar, bay
leaf, peppercorns and salt in a small non-stick saucepan over
a medium heat and bring to a simmer. Boil until the liquid has
reduced to just 2 tablespoons. Remove from the heat and
strain through a fine sieve into a small bowl.

Mix 2 tablespoons of the milk with the cornflour to form
a smooth paste. Pour the rest of the milk into a non-stick
saucepan and add the butter and the cornflour mixture. Bring
to a gentle simmer and cook for 2 minutes, stirring constantly
until smooth and thick.

Stir in the vinegar reduction and the tarragon. Cook very
gently over a low heat for 2 minutes. Beat the egg yolks
in a heatproof bowl until light and pale. Pour the eggs over
the hot milk, stirring continuously for 1–2 minutes. Adjust
the seasoning to taste. Remove from the heat and cover
to keep the sauce warm.

Trim any hard fat from the beef and season well with the
pepper and salt. Spray or brush a large non-stick frying pan
with oil and place over a medium-high heat. Add the steaks
and fry for 2½–3 minutes on each side or until done to taste.

Serve the steaks with the warm Béarnaise sauce, chips and
a large mixed salad.

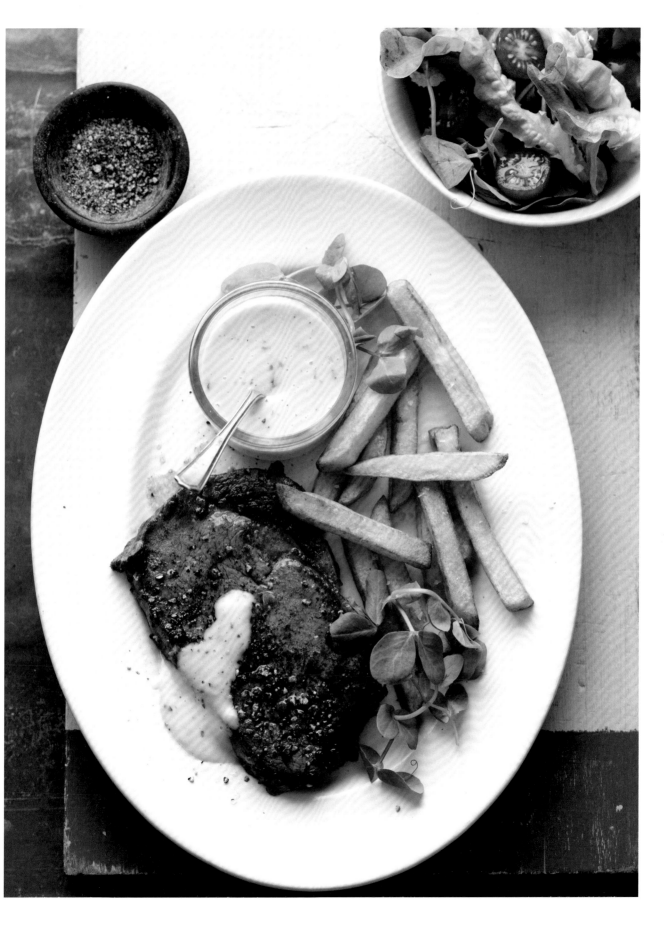

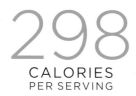

somerset pork and apples

SERVES 4
PREP: 15 MINUTES
COOK: 12 MINUTES

500g pork tenderloin (fillet)
1 tbsp sunflower oil
15g butter
2 small red eating apples,
   quartered, cored and sliced
1 medium onion, cut into
   12 wedges
2 tbsp cornflour
2 tbsp cold water
250ml dry cider
150ml pork stock (made
   with ½ pork stock cube)
1 tsp soft light brown sugar
3 tbsp half-fat crème fraiche
6–8 fresh sage leaves,
   thinly sliced
flaked sea salt
ground black pepper

Pork tenderloin (or fillet) is naturally lean and when cooked quickly, it will remain juicy and tender. This dish has a delicious cider sauce with apples. Serve with a small portion of boiled or mashed potatoes and lots of freshly cooked green vegetables.

Trim the pork of any fat or sinew and cut into 1.5cm slices. Season well with salt and pepper. Heat half the oil in a large non-stick frying pan over a high heat.

Fry the pork for about 2 minutes until nicely coloured on both sides but not completely cooked. Transfer it to a plate. Add the butter to the frying pan and return the pan to the heat. Stir-fry the apples for about 2 minutes until golden, then transfer them to a separate plate.

Tip the onion and remaining oil into the same pan and cook over a medium heat for 2–3 minutes, stirring occasionally until lightly browned. Mix the cornflour with the cold water in a small bowl until smooth.

Stir the cider, stock and sugar into the pan with the onion and bring to a simmer over a high heat. Cook for 2 minutes. Stir in the cornflour mixture and add the crème fraiche and sage.

Return the pork and any resting juices to the pan and simmer for 2 minutes or until cooked through, adding the apples for the last minute or so of the cooking time.

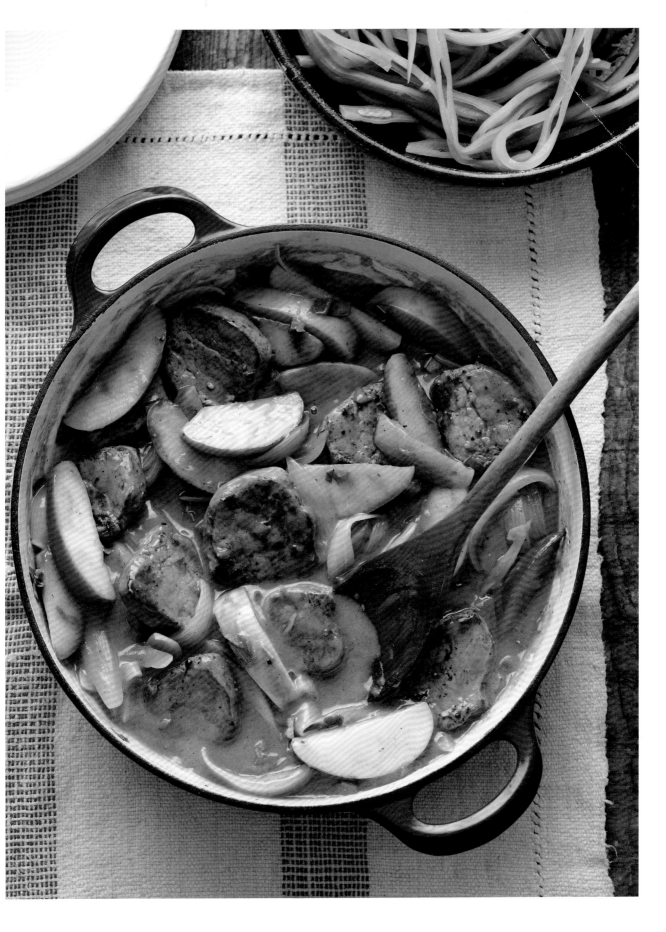

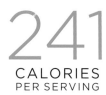

241
CALORIES
PER SERVING

spiced mango pork steaks

SERVES 4
PREP: 5 MINUTES
COOK: 12 MINUTES

1 tbsp sunflower oil
1 tsp ground coriander
1 tsp ground cumin
½ tsp hot chilli powder
½ tsp ground turmeric
2 tbsp mango chutney
4 boneless lean pork
   loin steaks (each
   about 150g)

A quick, spicy way to serve pork that might otherwise be a little dull. I trim most of the fat from each pork steak, leaving just enough to add flavour. Serve with a small portion of rice or some new potatoes and a large salad or green vegetables. A spoonful or two of fat-free natural yoghurt is a nice addition served on the side.

Pour the oil into a large mixing bowl and stir in the coriander, cumin, chilli powder and turmeric until thoroughly combined. Add the mango chutney to the spice mixture and stir well.

Preheat the grill to its hottest setting. Trim the pork of most of the hard fat. Turn the pork steaks in the spice mix until lightly coated. (Reserve the remaining spice mixture.)

Place the chops on a rack over a foil-lined grill pan. Cook for about 5 minutes on each side, then turn over once more and brush thickly with the remaining spice and mango mixture. Return to the grill for a further 2 minutes or until the pork is cooked through and the basting sauce is glossy and browned in places.

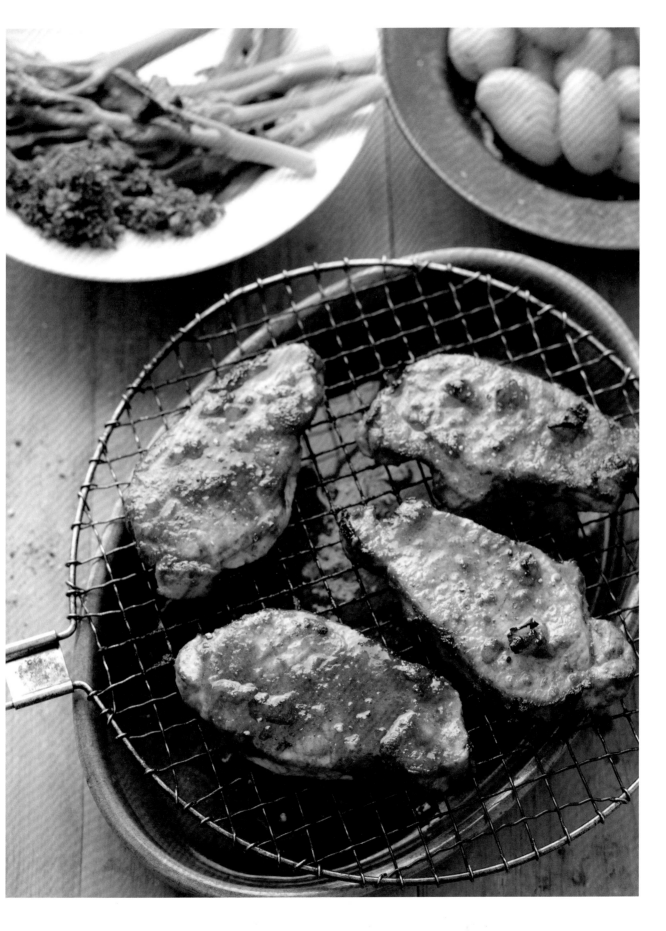

286 CALORIES PER SERVING

skewerless lamb kebabs

SERVES 4

PREP: 10 MINUTES, PLUS MARINATING

COOK: 20 MINUTES

500g lean lamb leg steaks or boneless lamb leg meat

3 mixed colour peppers, deseeded and cut into roughly 2.5cm chunks

2 medium red onions, each cut into 8 wedges

FOR THE MARINADE

freshly squeezed juice of 1 large lemon (about 4 tbsp)

2 garlic cloves, crushed

½ tsp cayenne pepper

1 tsp ground cumin

1 tbsp olive oil

½ tsp flaked sea salt

1 tsp coarsely ground black pepper

TO SERVE

100ml fat-free natural yoghurt

3 little gem lettuces, leaves separated

lemon wedges, for squeezing

fresh coriander or mint leaves, to garnish (optional)

A good lamb shish kebab can make a delicious meal, but the combination of fatty lamb and huge pitta wraps create a high calorie choice. My recipe uses lean lamb, simply marinated and stir-fried, so there is no fiddling around with skewers. Serve with little gem lettuce leaves instead of pitta to hold the meat and vegetables and you'll save up to 190 calories.

Trim the lamb of any hard fat, then cut the meat into roughly 2.5cm chunks and put in a large bowl. Add all the marinade ingredients and toss well together. Leave to stand for 15 minutes (or you can leave to marinate in the fridge for up to 2 hours before cooking if you like).

Place a large non-stick frying pan or wok over a high heat and drain the lamb from the marinade in a sieve. Cook the lamb in two batches for about 5 minutes or until well browned but not cooked through. Turn occasionally and only when you are sure the lamb is nicely browned on the side closest to the pan. Transfer to a plate between batches.

Add the peppers and onions to the pan and stir-fry for a further 3–4 minutes until softened and lightly charred.

Return the lamb and any resting juices to the pan and cook for a further 2 minutes until the lamb is just cooked – it should be pale pink in the centre. If in doubt, take a piece from the pan and cut it in half.

Serve the lamb with yoghurt, little gem leaves for wrapping and lemon wedges for squeezing. Scatter with freshly chopped coriander or mint leaves if you like.

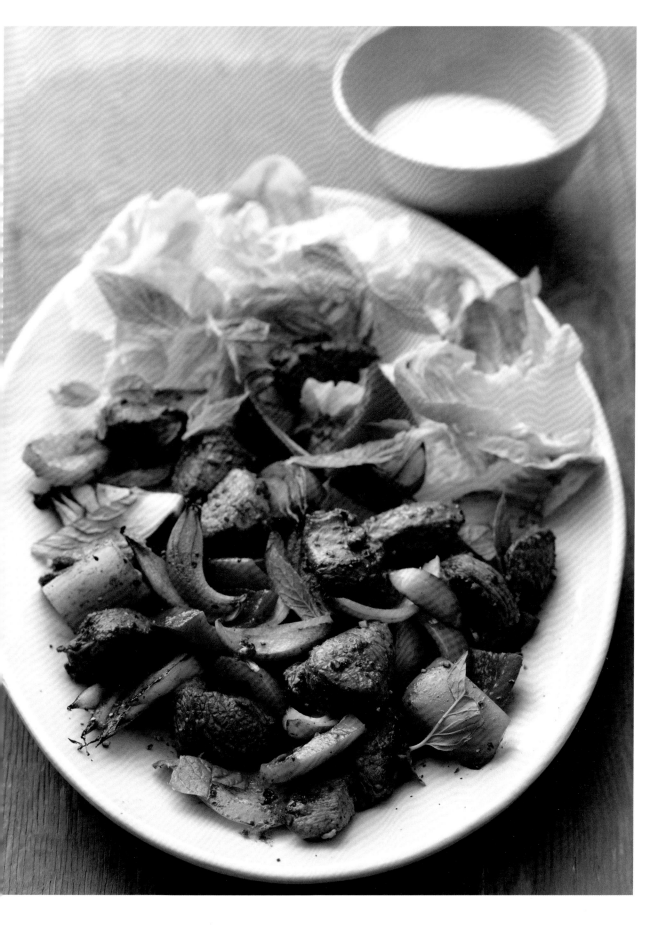

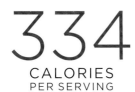

334 CALORIES PER SERVING

lamb cutlets with gremolata

SERVES 4
PREP: 10 MINUTES
COOK: 15 MINUTES

2 well-trimmed racks of
  lamb (each about 325g)
2 tsp sunflower oil
flaked sea salt
ground black pepper

FOR THE GREMOLATA
15g fresh parsley
15g fresh mint
finely grated zest of
  ½ lemon
1 small garlic clove,
  very finely chopped
2 tsp extra virgin olive oil

**For this recipe, look out for extra-trimmed racks of lamb –
all the fat has been trimmed off for you. One rack should
be just right for two people. Serve with a small portion
of new potatoes and a lightly dressed salad or freshly
cooked vegetables.**

Preheat the oven to 200°C/Fan 180°C/Gas 6. Season the lamb
on both sides really well with salt and pepper. Heat the sunflower
oil in a large non-stick frying pan and fry the lamb on all sides
for 2–3 minutes or until lightly browned. Put the lamb on a small
baking tray and roast in the oven for 10 minutes.

While the lamb is cooking, trim the parsley and mint and finely
chop the leaves. Put them in a bowl and stir in the lemon zest
and garlic. Take the lamb out of the oven and leave to rest for
5 minutes.

Carve the lamb into separate cutlets and put the cutlets on
a warmed platter. Scatter the gremolata over the top, drizzle
with the olive oil and season with a little more pepper.

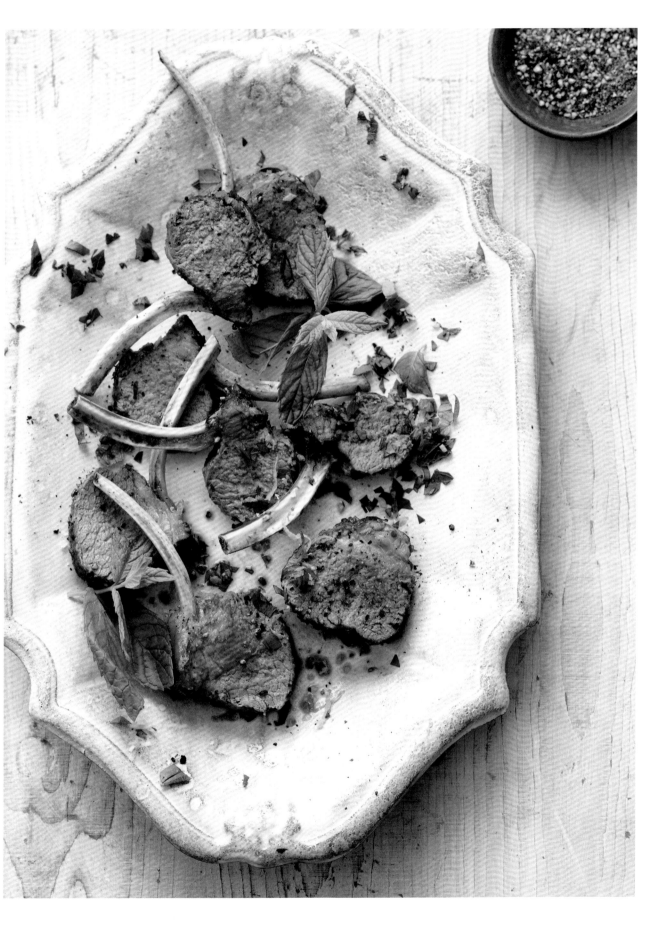

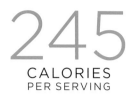

quick calzone

SERVES 4

PREP: 10 MINUTES

COOK: 10 MINUTES

400g can chopped
  tomatoes with herbs
2 tbsp tomato purée
4 large flour tortilla wraps
  (each about 60g)
50g prosciutto or wafer-
  thin ham (about 4 slices)
50g ready-grated
  mozzarella
20g fresh basil, leaves
  roughly torn
dried chilli flakes (optional)
ground black pepper

Freeze the folded calzone
before grilling and wrap
them tightly in foil. Freeze
for 1 month. Unwrap and
cook on a baking tray from
frozen in a preheated oven
at 200°C/Fan 180°C/Gas 6
for 10 minutes or until
lightly browned and hot
throughout. The calzones
can also be open frozen,
unfolded, then wrapped
in foil. Grill from frozen for
3–5 minutes until hot.

Based on my popular pizza pronto recipe in *Takeaway Favourites Without the Calories,* these folded pizzas lend themselves to being served with a salad on the side. You can also eat them folded and held in a wodge of paper napkins.

Preheat the grill to its hottest setting and place a large baking tray under the grill to warm. Put the tomatoes in a sieve and a shake gently over the sink a few times to drain most of the excess juice. Tip them into a bowl and mix with the tomato purée.

Place one of the tortillas on the warm baking tray and spread with a quarter of the tomatoes, leaving a 2cm gap around the edge.

Tear the prosciutto or ham into strips and arrange on top of the tomatoes. Sprinkle with the cheese and season with ground black pepper and chilli if you like.

Place under the hot grill for 1½–2½ minutes or until the cheese has melted and the edges of the pizza are beginning to brown.

Slide the pizza onto a board or warmed plate, top with a few basil leaves, fold over and serve with a colourful salad. Make the other calzone in the same way.

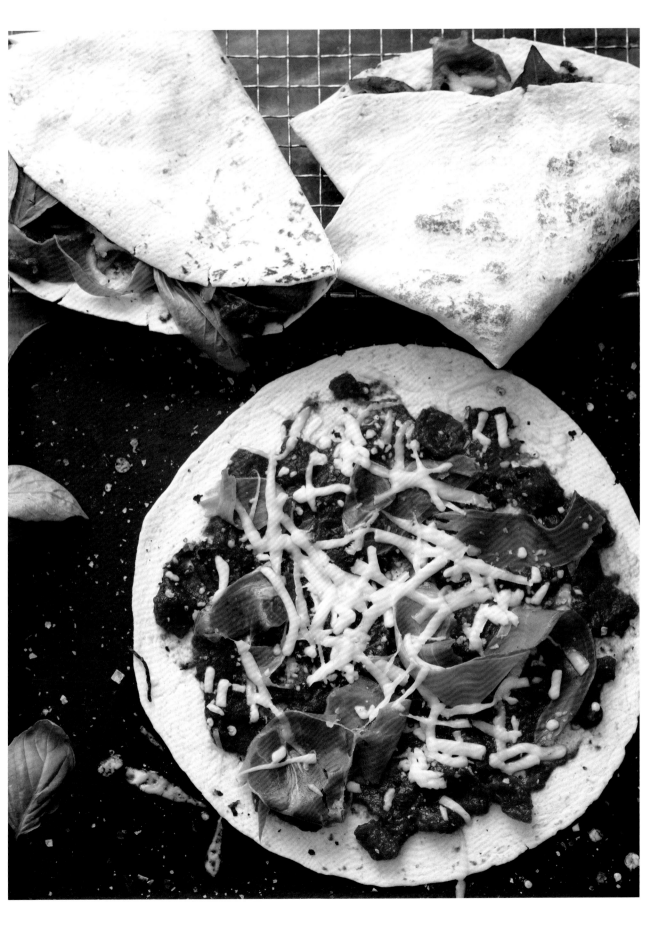

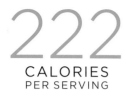

222
CALORIES
PER SERVING

beef stroganoff

SERVES 4

PREP: 10 MINUTES

COOK: 12 MINUTES

2 x 200g sirloin steaks
1 tbsp sunflower oil
250g chestnut mushrooms,
   sliced
2 medium onions, thinly
   sliced
1 tbsp plain flour
1 tsp paprika (not smoked)
300ml beef stock (made
   with 1 stock cube)
3 tbsp half-fat crème fraiche
   or soured cream
flaked sea salt
ground black pepper
chopped flat-leaf parsley,
   to garnish (optional)

This beef stroganoff has a rich, flavoursome sauce rather than the dull, grey version so often seen in low-calorie cookbooks. It contains lots of mushrooms and onions that make it extra filling too. Serve with small portions of rice or tagliatelle.

Trim the steak of all hard fat and thinly slice the meat on a slight diagonal into long strips around 5mm thick. Season well with salt and lots of freshly ground black pepper.

Heat a teaspoon of oil in a large non-stick frying pan or wok and stir-fry the steak strips over a high heat for 1–2 minutes until nicely browned but not cooked through. Transfer to a plate.

Add the rest of the oil, the mushrooms and onions to the pan and cook for 5 minutes until softened and well browned, stirring often.

Stir in the flour and paprika then gradually add the stock. Bring to the boil, stirring continuously. Reduce the heat slightly and simmer for 3 minutes.

Add the crème fraiche or soured cream, then return the beef with any resting juices to the pan and cook for a few seconds more until hot, stirring continuously. Scatter with the fresh parsley, if using, just before serving.

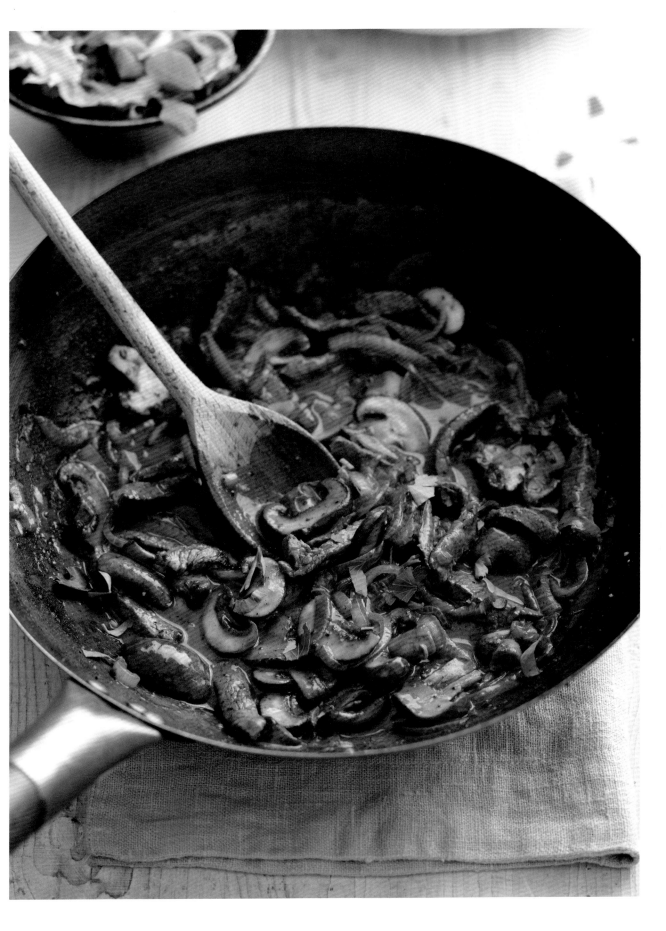

227
CALORIES
PER SERVING

balsamic steak with white bean mash

SERVES 2
PREP: 5 MINUTES
COOK: 6-8 MINUTES

2 x 150g fillet steaks
oil, for spraying or brushing
½ tsp flaked sea salt, plus extra for seasoning
1 tsp coarsely ground black pepper, plus extra for seasoning
100g baby button mushrooms, halved or quartered if large
125g cherry tomatoes, halved
2 tbsp thick balsamic vinegar
2 tbsp cold water
flaked sea salt
white bean mash (see right), to serve

I always keep a bottle of thick, good quality balsamic vinegar in my kitchen. It makes a great low-fat dressing dribbled over salad leaves and is brilliant for livening up meat dishes. It is pricey, but a little goes a long way.

Trim any hard fat from the beef. Season the steaks well with the salt and the pepper.

Spray or brush a large non-stick frying pan with oil and place over a medium-high heat. Add the steaks and fry for 3–4 minutes on each side or until done to taste (around 3 minutes on each side will give a rare steak but you may need to cook for 5–6 minutes on each side if you prefer well done steak, depending on the thickness).

Add the mushrooms and tomatoes to the pan after 3 minutes, or once the steaks have been turned, and cook until the mushrooms are lightly browned and the tomatoes are softened, stirring occasionally.

Remove the pan from the heat and transfer the steaks to two warmed plates. Pour the vinegar and water into the hot pan, off the heat, and bubble for a few seconds, stirring to lift any juicy bits from the bottom. Pour over the steaks and serve with my everyday salad (see page 30) or any green salad.

White bean mash: Drain and rinse 2 x 400g cans of butter beans or cannellini beans and put them in a food processor with ½ crushed garlic clove, 6 tablespoons cold water, ½ teaspoon flaked sea salt and a few twists of ground black pepper. Blitz until smooth, pushing the mixture down with a spatula if necessary. Put the mash in a small saucepan and heat gently, stirring constantly until hot. Drizzle with a teaspoon of extra virgin olive oil before serving. Serves 2. Calories per serving: 199

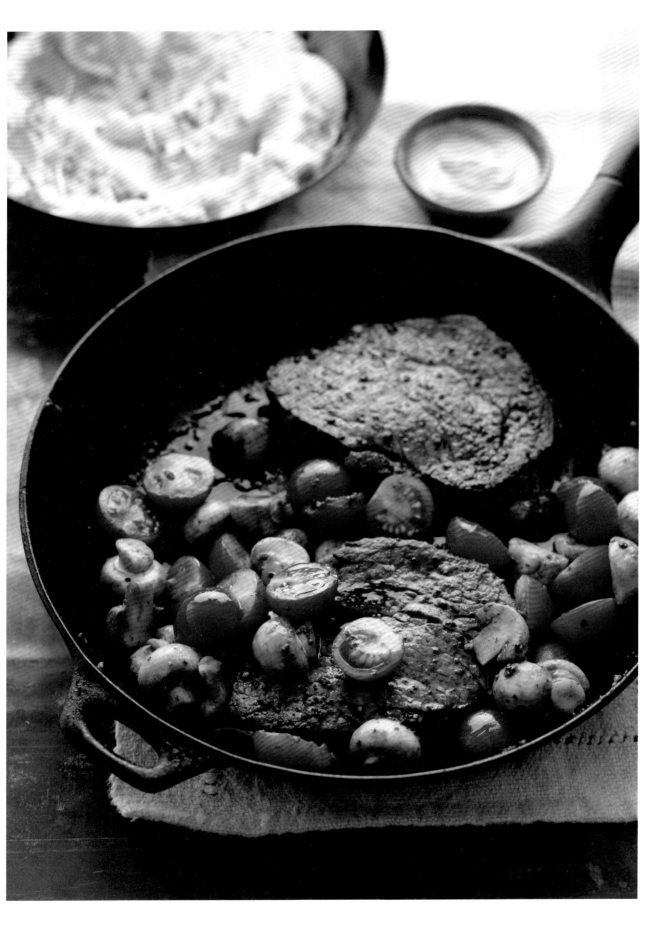

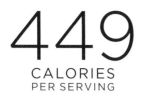

449
CALORIES
PER SERVING

mozzarella meatballs lasagne

SERVES 4
PREP 10 MINUTES
COOK 40 MINUTES

24 small lean beef meatballs (about 400g)
6 sheets no-precook dried egg lasagne (about 110g)
50g ready-grated mozzarella

FOR THE SAUCE
oil, for spraying or brushing
1 medium onion, coarsely grated
2 x 400g cans chopped tomatoes
2 tbsp tomato purèe
350ml beef stock (made with 1 beef stock cube)
100ml red wine or extra stock
1 tsp dried oregano
flaked sea salt
ground black pepper

Freeze the cooled unbaked lasagne covered tightly with foil for up to 2 months. Thaw overnight in the fridge and reheat as the recipe for about 30 minutes, removing the foil for the last 10 minutes of cooking time until piping hot throughout.

You don't have to cook the pasta or make the meatballs for this easy to prepare and generous lasagne. If you can't get small meatballs, use larger ones and cut them in half or make your own with 400g lean minced beef.

Preheat the oven to 200°C/Fan 180°C/Gas 6. To make the sauce, spray or brush a wide-based saucepan or sauté pan with oil and fry the onion gently for 5 minutes or until softened, stirring regularly.

Add the tomatoes to the pan and stir in the tomato purèe, stock, wine, if using, and oregano. Bring to a gentle simmer and cook uncovered for 15 minutes, stirring occasionally.

While the sauce is simmering, brush a large baking tray lightly with oil and arrange the meatballs. Bake for 10 minutes or until lightly browned on all sides.

Add the meatballs to the pan with the tomatoes and cook for 10 minutes more, stirring occasionally until the meatballs are cooked through and the sauce is rich and thick.

Meanwhile, half fill a large saucepan with water and bring to the boil. Add the lasagne sheets one at a time and return to the boil. Cook for 7 minutes or until tender, stirring occasionally to stop the lasagne sticking together. Drain in a colander.

Take the meatballs and sauce off the heat. Add the lasagne and mix lightly. Tumble the lasagne and meatball sauce into a large, warmed lasagne dish. Pull up a few of the lasagne sheets with a fork. Sprinkle with the cheese and bake for 10 minutes or until the cheese melts and the sauce begins to bubble.

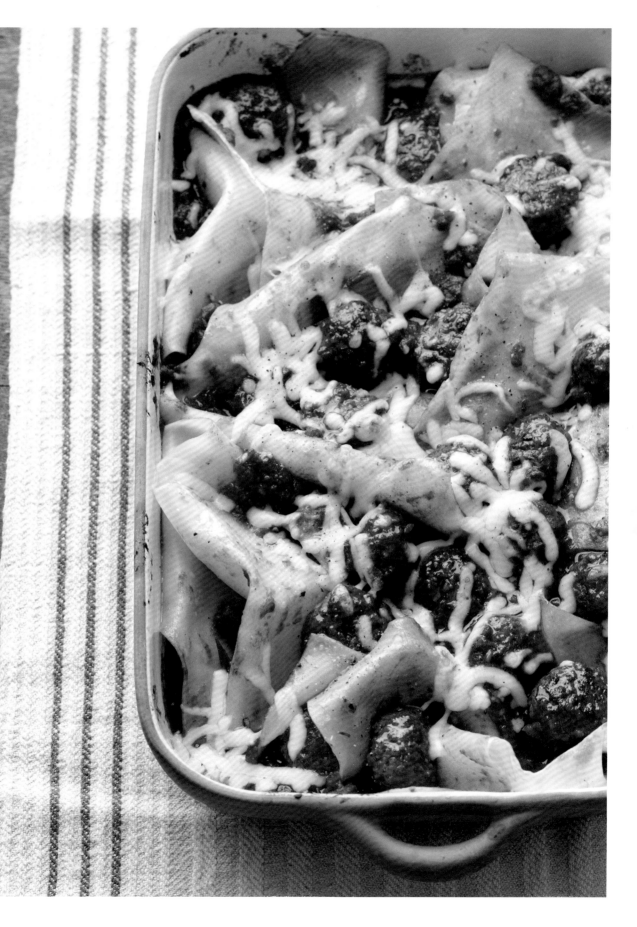

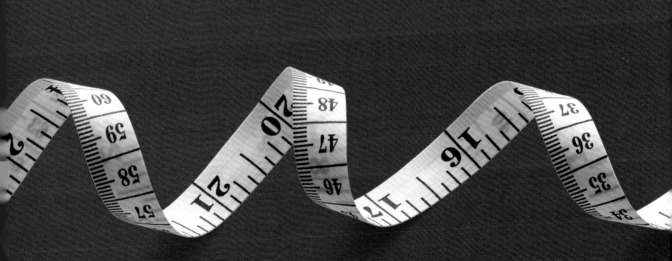

fish and
seafood

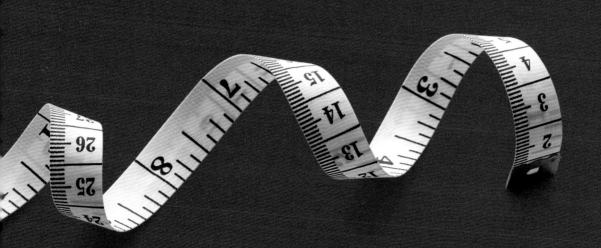

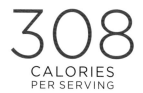

308
CALORIES
PER SERVING

salmon provençal

SERVES 4

PREP: 10 MINUTES

COOK: 35 MINUTES

1 medium red onion,
  cut into 12 wedges
1 red and 1 yellow pepper,
  deseeded and cut into
  roughly 3cm chunks
2 medium courgettes, cut
  into roughly 1.5cm slices
1 tbsp extra virgin olive oil
4 x 125g skinless salmon
  fillets
300g cherry tomatoes
  on the vine, snipped
  into short lengths
1 tbsp thick balsamic
  vinegar
15g fresh basil leaves,
  roughly torn
flaked sea salt
ground black pepper

It's worth making this quantity even if you are serving fewer than four, as the cold salmon and vegetables make a great salad for the next day. To cut the calories even further, spray rather than dribble the oil on your vegetables or use white fish fillet.

Preheat the oven to 220°C/Fan 200°C/Gas 7. Put the onion, peppers and courgettes in a large roasting tin, dribble over the oil and season with salt and pepper. Toss lightly together, then bake for 20 minutes.

Take the tin out of the oven and turn the vegetables. Make four spaces and nestle the salmon fillets into the tray. Add the cherry tomatoes and season with black pepper.

Bake for a further 15 minutes or until the salmon is just cooked and the vegetables are tender and lightly charred. Drizzle with the balsamic vinegar and scatter the basil leaves over just before serving.

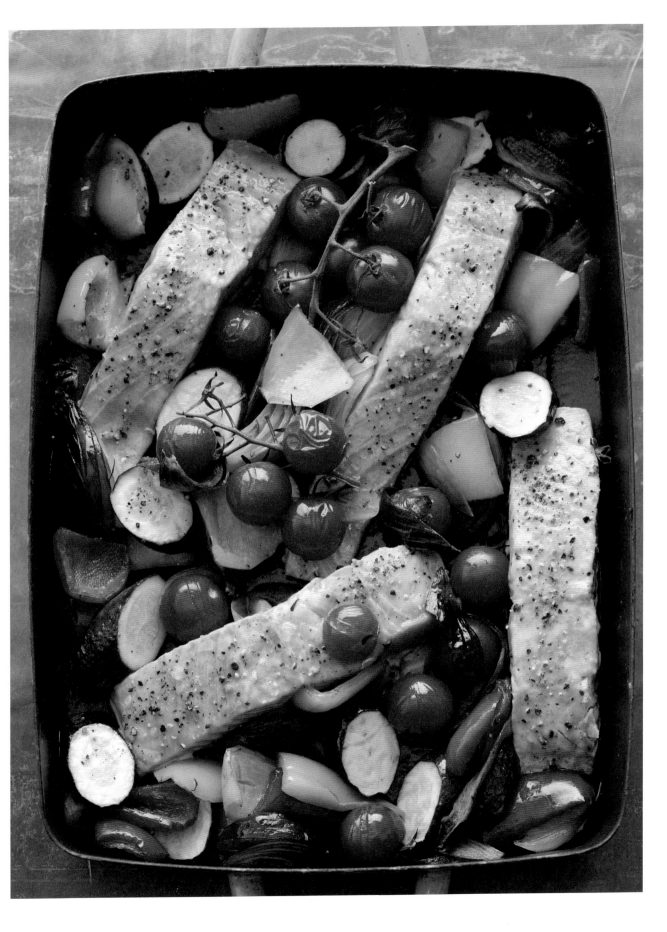

199
CALORIES
PER SERVING

pan-fried cod with asian dressing

SERVES 2
PREP: 5 MINUTES
COOK: 10 MINUTES

2 tbsp fresh lime juice
1 tbsp Thai fish sauce
   (nam pla)
1 tbsp soft light brown sugar
½ tsp dried chilli flakes
oil, for spraying or brushing
2 x 150g thick white fish
   fillets, such as cod or
   haddock, with skin
lime wedges, for squeezing
flaked sea salt
ground black pepper

MIXED VEGETABLES
100g mangetout
100g long-stemmed
   broccoli, cut in half
1 medium leek, thinly sliced

Plainly cooked fish can be a little dull, but this zingy Asian-inspired dressing really brings this dish to life. You can serve with small portions of rice, but I think it's perfect just as it is.

To make the dressing, mix the lime juice, fish sauce, brown sugar and chilli in a small bowl and set aside.

Spray or brush a small frying pan with oil and place over a high heat. Season the fish all over with salt and pepper. Cook the fish, skin-side down, for 3 minutes or until the skin is crisp. Turn the fish over, reduce the heat to low and cook for a further 3–5 minutes or until just cooked, depending on thickness. The centre of the fish will be creamy white rather than translucent when the fish is cooked.

While the fish is cooking, fill a medium pan a third full of water and bring it to the boil. Add the vegetables, return to the boil and cook for 2 minutes or until just tender. Drain in a colander and divide between warmed plates.

Top the vegetables with the fish and spoon over the dressing. Serve with lime wedges for squeezing.

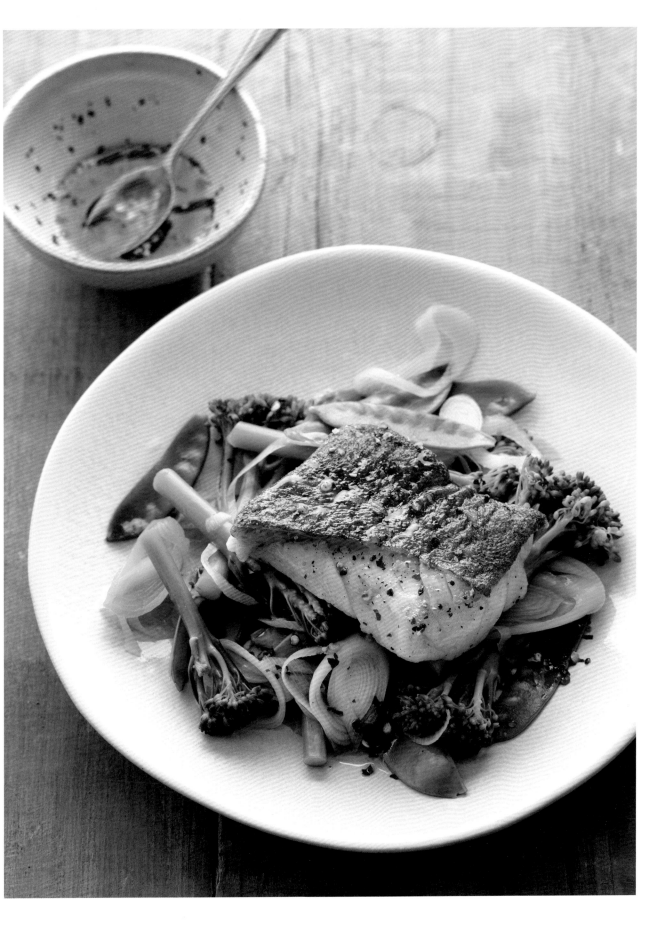

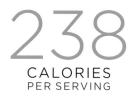

238
CALORIES
PER SERVING

fish sticks with lemony garlic mayo

SERVES 4
PREP: 20 MINUTES
COOK: 12 MINUTES

4 x 125g thin skinless fish
   fillets, such as plaice
   or sole
25g plain flour
good pinch of fine sea salt
1 large egg
100g dried coarse white
   breadcrumbs or
   panko breadcrumbs
½ tsp paprika (not smoked)
½ tsp ground turmeric
oil, for spraying
freshly ground black pepper
lemon wedges, for
   squeezing
lemony garlic mayo
   (see right), to serve

Open freeze the uncooked
but coated fish until solid
then pack into freezer-proof
containers, interleaving with
baking parchment for up
to 3 months. Cook as the
recipe, adding an extra
3-5 minutes, ensuring the
fish inside is cooked.

These delicious strips of crisp fish can be prepared ahead
and then frozen until you need them. The turmeric and paprika
colour the breadcrumbs and give the fish sticks a golden
brown crumb even though they aren't fried. Serve with lemony
garlic mayo (see below) or tomato ketchup for dipping.

Preheat the oven to 200°C/Fan 180°C/Gas 6. Put the fish
on a board and cut each fillet into 2cm-wide strips at a slight
diagonal angle from one end to the other.

Put the flour in a bowl and season with the salt and some
pepper. Beat the egg in a medium bowl with a metal whisk
until smooth. Sprinkle half the breadcrumbs, half the paprika
and half the turmeric into a large bowl.

Toss the fish pieces with the seasoned flour. Take one at a time
and dip each piece into the beaten egg and then coat in the
breadcrumbs until evenly covered.

Put the pieces on a tray lined with baking parchment while y
ou prepare the rest, adding the reserved breadcrumbs, paprika
and turmeric to the large bowl after coating roughly half the
fish pieces. Spray all the fish with oil and bake for 12 minutes
until golden and crisp.

Lemony garlic mayo: Mix 4 tablespoons light mayonnaise,
4 tablespoons fat-free yoghurt, 1 small crushed garlic clove
and finely grated zest of ½ lemon in a small serving bowl.
Serves 4. Calories per serving: 52

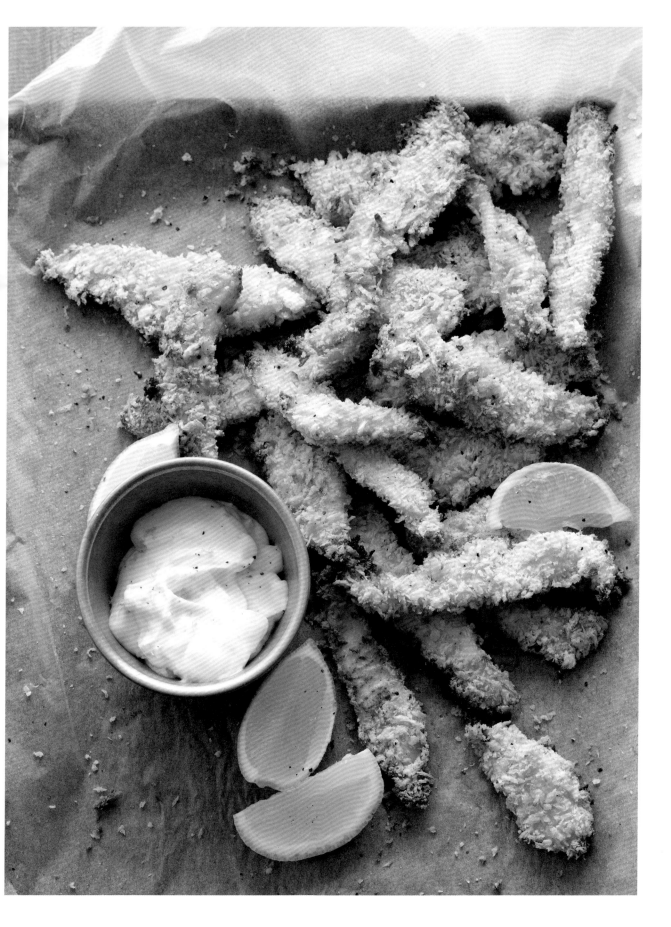

283

CALORIES
PER SERVING

fresh tuna niçoise

SERVES 4

PREP: 5 MINUTES

COOK: 15 MINUTES

200g fine green beans,
   trimmed
4 fridge-cold eggs
2 x 150g very fresh
   tuna steaks
4 little gem lettuces,
   leaves separated
1 small red onion,
   thinly sliced
50g pitted black olives,
   drained (about 20 olives)
1 tsp sunflower oil
4 tbsp reduced-calorie
   Caesar dressing
flaked sea salt
freshly ground black pepper

A lovely, summery salad. If you don't fancy using fresh tuna, use 2 x 120g cans of tuna steak in water, or a couple of griddled chicken breasts instead. The salad is also good with a small serving of new potatoes, but just as filling without.

Fill a medium saucepan a third full of water and bring to the boil. Add the green beans, return to the boil and cook for 2–3 minutes or until they are just tender. Drain in a colander under running water until cold.

Half fill the same saucepan with water and bring it to the boil. Gently add the eggs to the pan with a slotted spoon and boil for 8 minutes. Drain in a sieve under running water until cool enough to handle, then peel and quarter them.

Meanwhile, season the tuna steaks with salt and plenty of freshly ground black pepper. Roughly tear the lettuce leaves and put them in a large serving bowl or platter and add the red onion, drained green beans and the olives.

Heat the oil in a large non-stick frying pan over a medium-high heat. Add the tuna steaks and cook for 1½–2 minutes on each side, until lightly browned but slightly pink in the middle, or until done to taste.

Arrange the eggs on top of the salad. Break the warm tuna steaks into large chunks and drop gently on top. Drizzle with the Caesar dressing and serve.

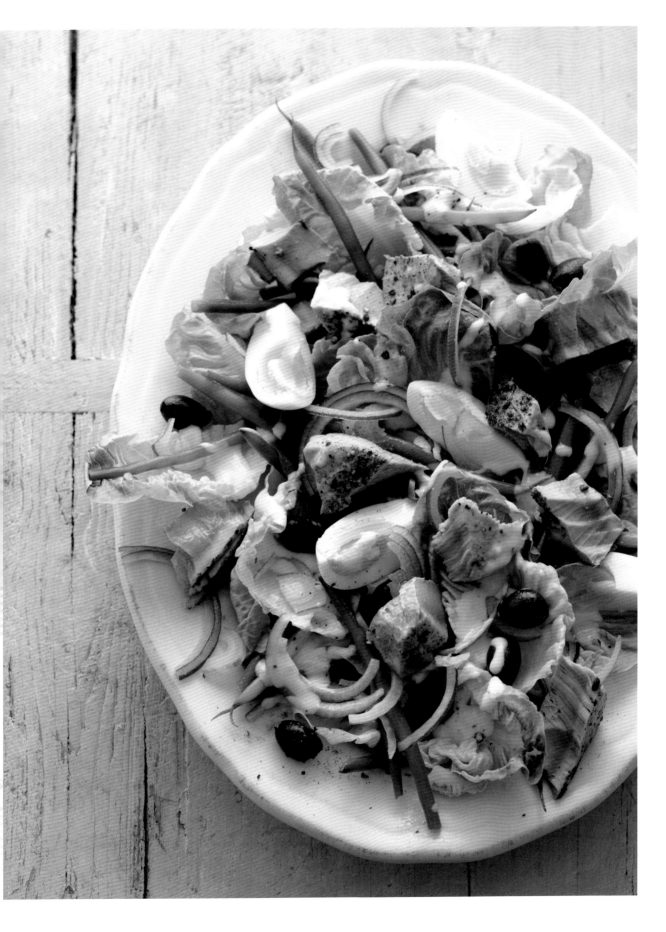

139 CALORIES PER SERVING

tuna and bean salad

SERVES 4

PREP: 10 MINUTES

2 x 120g cans tuna steak
  in water or brine, drained
400g can cannellini beans,
  drained and rinsed
½ small red onion, thinly
  sliced
1 red pepper, deseeded
  and cut into roughly
  2cm chunks
¼ cucumber, cut into
  roughly 2cm dice
12 pitted black or green
  olives, drained and halved
  (optional)
100g cherry tomatoes,
  halved
15g flat-leaf parsley, leaves
  roughly chopped
1–2 tbsp thick balsamic
  vinegar
ground black pepper

Tip: Add 200g cooked
pasta shapes to the salad
for roughly an extra 80
calories per serving.

Packing a lunch for work can be tricky when you are hoping to lose weight, but this simple salad can be quickly assembled in the morning and is robust enough to last until lunchtime.

Tip the tuna into a bowl and flake into chunky pieces with a fork. Scatter the beans into the same bowl and add the onion, pepper, cucumber, olives (if using), cherry tomatoes and parsley.

Toss all the ingredients lightly, divide between four plates or transfer to small, lidded containers and keep chilled until ready to eat. Drizzle with balsamic vinegar and season with freshly ground black pepper.

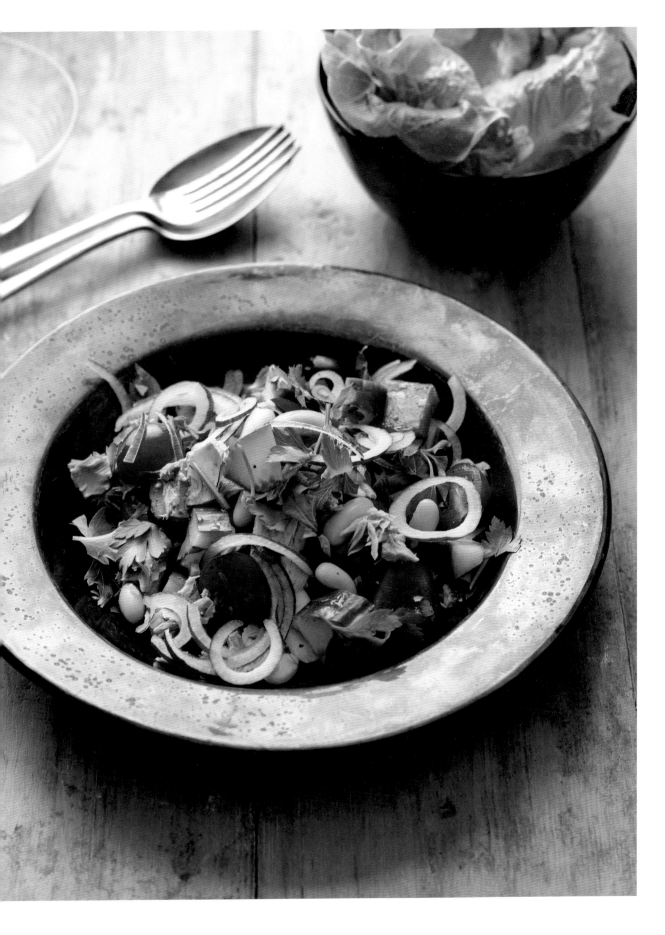

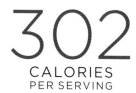

302 CALORIES PER SERVING

spanish prawns with rice

SERVES 5

PREP: 10 MINUTES

COOK: 25 MINUTES

oil, for spraying or brushing
100g soft cooking chorizo,
    cut into 5mm slices
2 medium onions, chopped
4 celery sticks, cut into
    roughly 1cm slices
2 mixed colour peppers,
    deseeded and cut into
    roughly 2cm chunks
2 large garlic cloves,
    crushed
1 tbsp paprika (not smoked)
½–1 tsp hot smoked paprika,
    depending on taste
175g easy-cook long
    grain rice
650ml chicken stock (made
    with 1 chicken stock cube)
350g cooked peeled
    prawns, thawed if frozen
flaked sea salt
ground black pepper
finely chopped fresh
    parsley, to garnish
    (optional)

Spanish chorizo sausage is high in fat, but the delicious smoky flavour really pulls through, so you shouldn't need too much of it. This prawn and rice one pan dish can be made in just over 30 minutes and will feed five people.

Spray or brush a large non-stick sauté pan or shallow flameproof casserole with the oil and place over a medium heat. Add the chorizo, onions, celery and peppers and cook for 5 minutes, stirring occasionally.

Add the garlic and sprinkle over the paprika, smoked paprika and rice. Stir well together. Pour over the chicken stock, season with a pinch of salt and lots of freshly ground black pepper.

Bring to a simmer and cook without covering for around 12–15 minutes or until the rice is tender and most of the liquid has been absorbed, stirring frequently towards the end of the cooking time to prevent the rice sticking.

Stir in the prawns and cook for 2–3 minutes more or until the prawns are hot, stirring regularly. Adjust seasoning to taste and garnish with fresh parsley if you like.

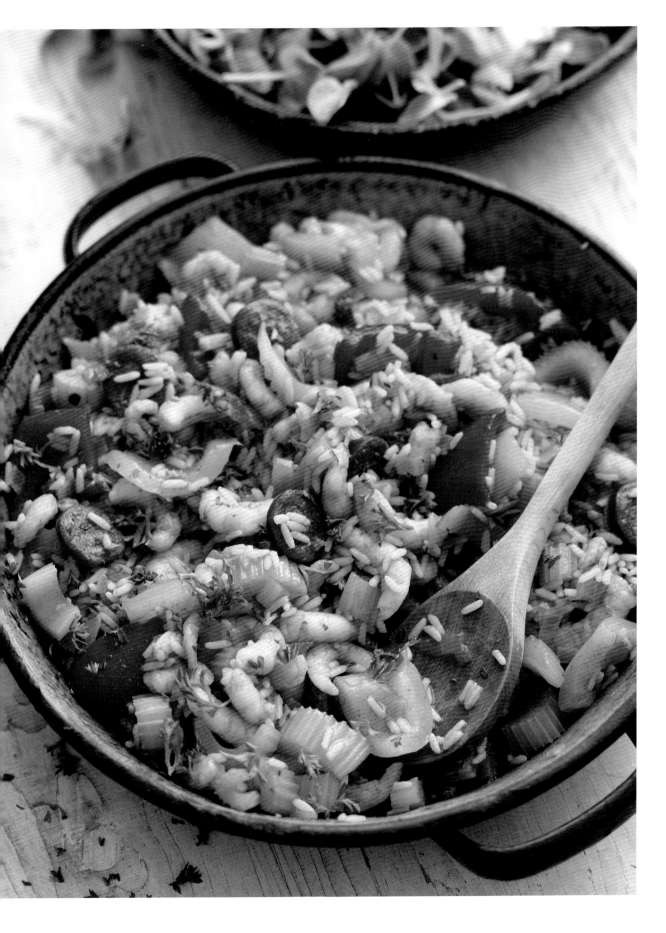

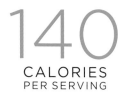

140
CALORIES
PER SERVING

spicy seasoned fish

SERVES 2
PREP: 5 MINUTES
COOK: 10 MINUTES

2 tbsp plain flour
2 tsp Creole or Cajun
  seasoning (from a jar)
¼ tsp flaked sea salt
¼ tsp freshly ground
  black pepper
oil, for spraying or brushing
2 x 125g thin fish fillets,
  such as plaice or sole
  (not skinned)
roughly chopped fresh
  coriander, to garnish
lemon or lime wedges,
  for squeezing

This is a great dish for anyone who doesn't usually cook fish as it's very simple – using seasoning from a jar – and incredibly quick to fry. Serve with a small portion of oven chips (5% or less fat) and a big, crunchy salad.

Mix the flour with the Creole or Cajun seasoning, salt and pepper in a large freezer bag. Take the fish fillets and drop them into the bag; toss until lightly coated with the seasoned flour.

Spray or brush a large non-stick frying pan with oil. Pat off the excess flour and fry the fish, one at a time, over a medium heat skin-side up for about 2½ minutes. Turn over and cook on the other side for about 2 minutes or until cooked through. Turn very gently or the fish could break up.

Serve hot, garnished with chopped coriander and with lemon or lime wedges to squeeze over the fish.

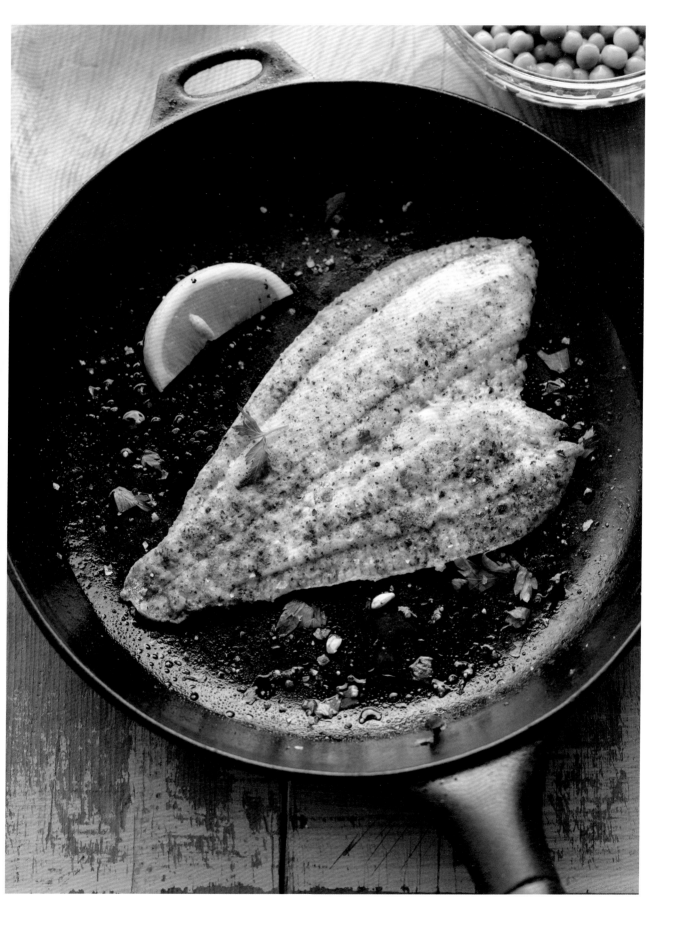

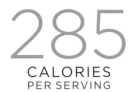

285
CALORIES
PER SERVING

chilli lemon prawns with tomato and broccoli spaghetti

SERVES 2

PREP: 5 MINUTES

COOK: 15 MINUTES

150g long-stemmed broccoli
80g dried spaghetti
200g cooked and peeled prawns, thawed if frozen
100g cherry tomatoes, halved
1 tbsp fresh lemon juice
1 tsp chilli oil
1 tsp dried chilli flakes
flaked sea salt
ground black pepper

A light summery dish that takes around 20 minutes from start to finish to prepare. Use any cooked prawns you like. The smaller, cold water prawns will have more flavour than warm water king prawns, but both work well in this dish. The spaghetti portion may seem small, but the vegetables will help fill you up.

Half fill a large saucepan with water and bring to the boil. Trim the broccoli and cut each stem into 3 pieces, leaving the heads intact.

Add the spaghetti to the boiling water, return to the boil and cook for 10 minutes, stirring occasionally. Add the broccoli to the same pan and cook for 2 minutes or until just tender.

Drain the pasta and broccoli in a colander, then tip them back into the same pan or a large non-stick wok. Add the prawns, tomatoes, lemon juice, chilli oil and chilli flakes.

Stir-fry for 2 minutes, tossing regularly until the prawns are hot and the tomatoes are softened but still holding their shape. Season with salt and lots of freshly ground black pepper.

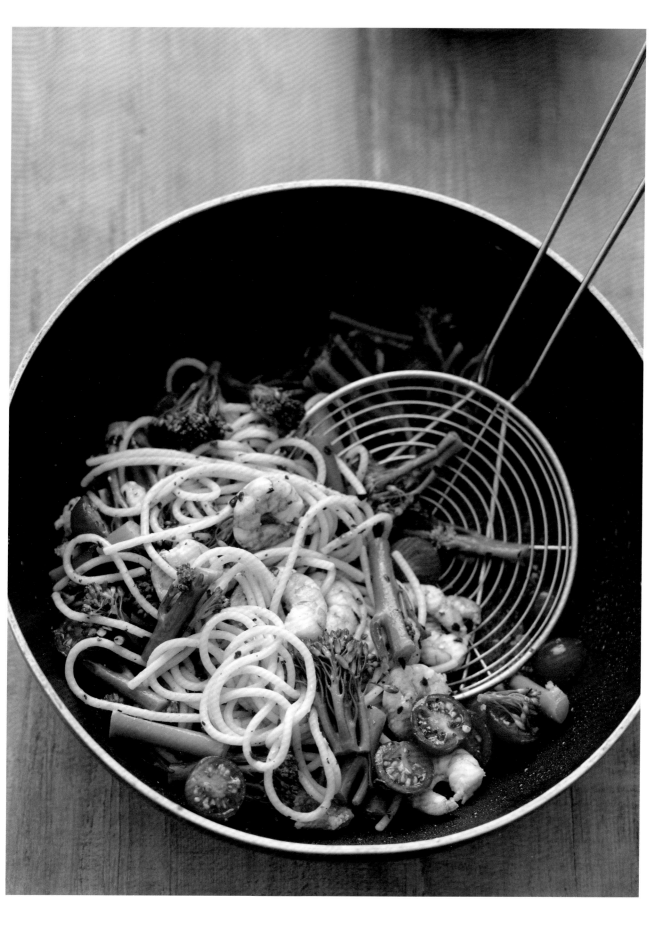

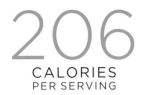

206
CALORIES
PER SERVING

tuna and sweetcorn cheat's jackets

SERVES 4

PREP: 5 MINUTES

COOK: 30 MINUTES

500g small new potatoes
oil, for spraying
120g can tuna steak in
    water or brine, drained
3 tbsp light mayonnaise
198g can sweetcorn, drained
4 spring onions, thinly sliced
flaked sea salt
ground black pepper

This is my take on the classic tuna mayonnaise filled jacket potato – something that can contain 475 calories or more. This recipe takes less than half the time to cook and is extra-delicious thanks to the crispy baked potato skins that make a nice contrast to the moist tuna and sweetcorn topping.

Fill a large pan one third full of water and bring it to the boil. Add the potatoes to the water and return to the boil. Cook for 15 minutes or until just tender.

Preheat the oven to 220°C/Fan 200°C/Gas 7. Drain the potatoes well in a colander. Spray a baking tray with oil. Tip the potatoes onto the tray and crush roughly with a spatula to break the skins and flatten them. Spray with oil and season with salt and lots of ground black pepper. Bake for 15 minutes or until the edges are crisp and golden.

While the potatoes are cooking, mix the tuna and mayonnaise, then lightly stir in the sweetcorn and spring onions.

Take the potatoes out of the oven and spoon the tuna mixture on top to serve.

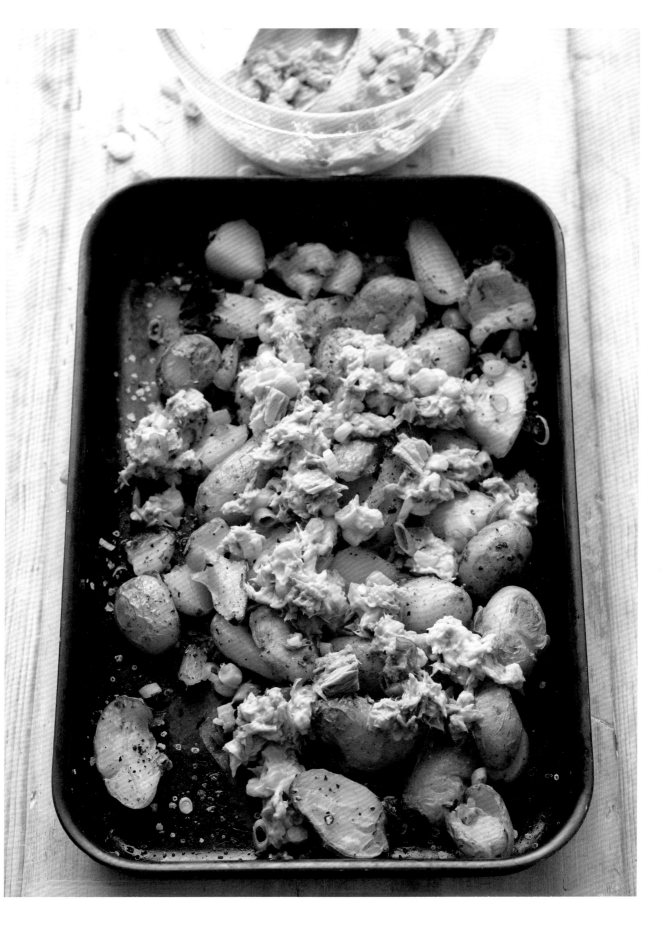

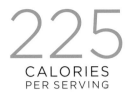

225
CALORIES
PER SERVING

prawn korma

A brilliant way of making a really creamy but low-calorie curry. This dish is lovely served with warm naan bread fingers or small portions of rice. If you don't want to use prawns, add chunks of white fish or cooked chicken pieces instead.

SERVES 4

PREP: 5 MINUTES

COOK: 15 MINUTES

2 medium onions, quartered
3 tbsp mild curry paste
200ml cold water,
   plus 3 tbsp
100ml fat-free natural
   yoghurt
2 tbsp mango chutney
400g cooked and peeled
   prawns, thawed if frozen
2 tbsp double cream
roughly chopped fresh
   coriander, to garnish
flaked sea salt
ground black pepper

Tip: Ready-made naan bread makes a quick and easy accompaniment to this curry. Simply heat as instructed on the packet for about 5 minutes and cut into fingers. Half a bought naan bread will add around 185 calories to your meal.

Put the onions and curry paste in a food processor and blitz until as smooth as possible. You may need to remove the lid and push the mixture down a couple of times until the right consistency is reached.

Tip the spiced puréed onions into a large, deep non-stick frying pan or wok and cook over a medium heat for 5 minutes, stirring regularly until they begin to soften. Add the 3 tablespoons of cold water and cook for a further 5 minutes or until the onions are well softened, stirring.

Pour over the remaining 200ml water and add the yoghurt and mango chutney. Bring to a gentle simmer and cook for 5 minutes or until the sauce is thick, stirring regularly. Add the prawns and double cream and cook for 1–2 minutes or until the prawns are heated through, stirring. Garnish with fresh coriander if you like.

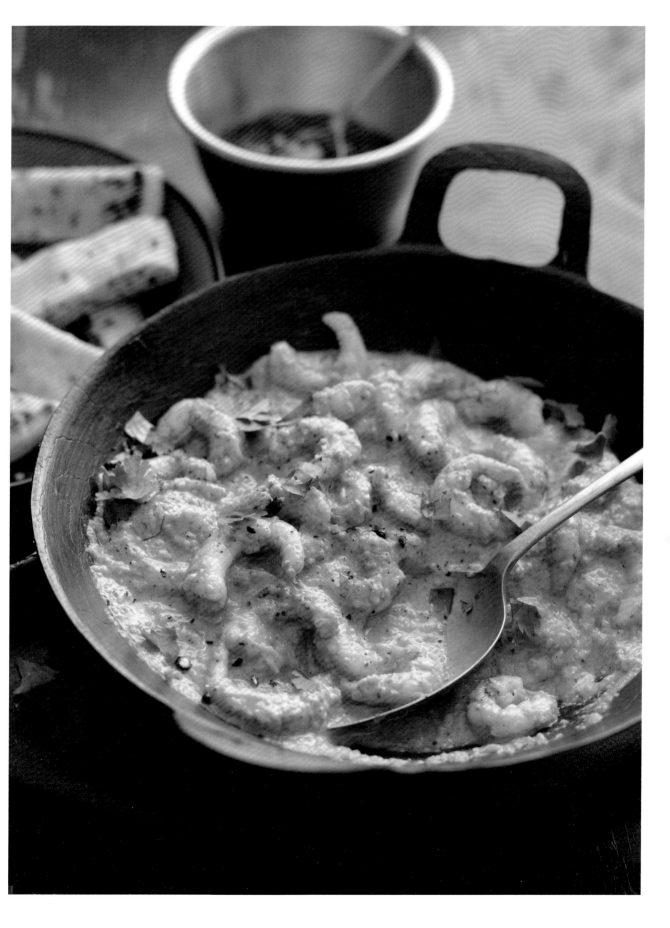

160
CALORIES
PER SERVING

fast cod in parsley sauce

SERVES 4

PREP: 10 MINUTES

COOK: 12 MINUTES

250ml semi-skimmed milk,
    plus 2 tbsp
½ small onion, thinly sliced
1 bay leaf
600g skinless white
    fish fillet, such as cod
    or haddock
15g fresh parsley, leaves
    finely chopped
1 tbsp cornflour
mashed potatoes
    (see below), to serve

Tip: Add a few prawns or
quartered hard-boiled eggs
to the fish and sauce for a
super-quick deconstructed
fish pie.

Chunky pieces of fish in a rich parsley sauce looks and tastes luxurious and is also low enough in calories for you to serve with a portion of mashed potatoes and stay right on track.

Put the milk in a saucepan and add the onion and bay leaf. Add a good pinch of salt and a little ground black pepper. Warm through gently for 5 minutes, stirring occasionally. Do not allow to boil. (Infusing the milk with onion will add flavour to the sauce.)

Cut the fish into roughly 4cm chunks and put in a large non-stick frying pan with the parsley. Strain the milk through a sieve onto the fish and place over a medium heat. Discard the onion and bay leaf.

Bring the milk to a gentle simmer without stirring. Mix the cornflour with the 2 tablespoons of milk until smooth and stir into the pan. Turn the fish pieces and simmer for about 3 minutes or until just cooked. Stir very gently as the sauce bubbles, and take care not to let the fish break up.

Adjust the seasoning to taste and serve the fish and parsley sauce with mashed potatoes and lots of fresh vegetables.

Mashed potatoes: Peel 500g potatoes and cut into roughly 3cm chunks. Put in a saucepan and cover with just-boiled water. Place over a high heat and bring to the boil. Reduce the heat to a fast simmer and cook for 10 minutes or until tender. Drain then return to the saucepan and mash with 15g butter, 5 tablespoons semi-skimmed milk, salt and pepper until smooth. Serves 4. Calories per serving: 130

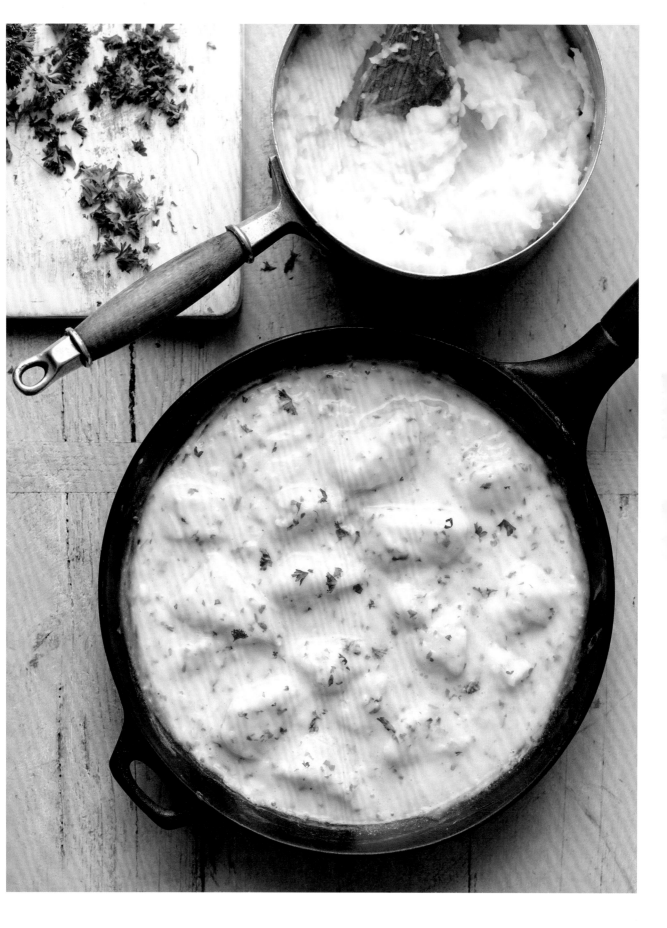

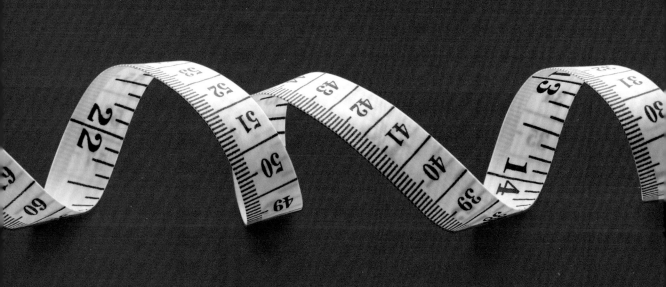

meat-free

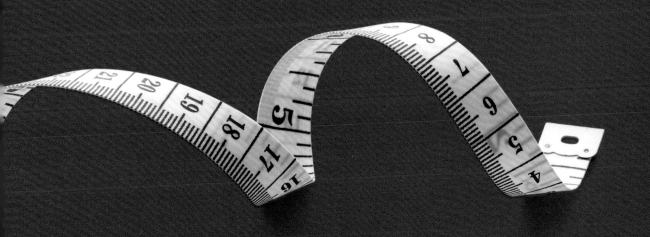

126
CALORIES
PER SERVING

tomato, ricotta and basil salad

SERVES 2

PREP: 10 MINUTES

300g mixed tomatoes,
    halved or quartered
    if large
100g ricotta cheese, drained
fresh basil leaves,
    roughly torn
2 tsp extra virgin olive oil
1 tsp thick balsamic vinegar
flaked sea salt
ground black pepper

This simple salad can be knocked together in no time and tastes deliciously light and fresh. You don't need to use different coloured tomatoes, but they do make it look very pretty. Ricotta is a medium-fat soft cheese with a very mild taste, so a dribble of thick balsamic vinegar adds a useful flavour kick.

Divide the tomatoes between two plates and top with the ricotta cheese, broken into pieces. Scatter basil leaves over the top and drizzle with olive oil. Season with salt and pepper. Drizzle with balsamic vinegar just before serving.

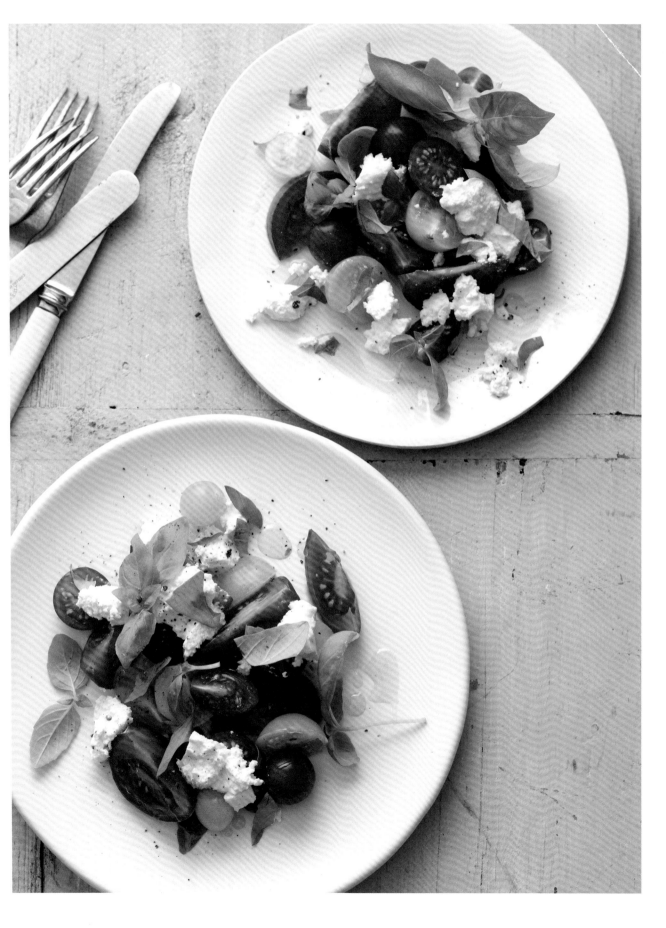

198
CALORIES
PER SERVING

spiced courgette fritters

SERVES 2
PREP: 10 MINUTES
COOK: 12 MINUTES

1 large courgette
  (about 265g)
3 tbsp plain flour
1 tsp ground cumin
1 tsp ground coriander
1 tsp flaked sea salt
1 egg, beaten
100g ricotta cheese, drained
oil, for spraying or brushing

These lightly spiced ricotta and courgette fritters are lovely served with a salad and yoghurt for lunch or as a simple snack. This recipe makes enough for two people as part of a light meal or four as a snack. They can be kept in the fridge for up to two days and then reheated in a pan over a low heat.

Trim and finely grate the courgette. Squeeze the excess water from the courgette with your hands over the sink.

Mix the flour, cumin, coriander and salt in a bowl. Add the grated courgette and stir well. Tip the beaten egg and ricotta into the bowl and mix until well combined.

Spray a large non-stick frying pan with oil and place over a low heat. Gently drop 5–6 large spoonfuls of batter into the pan, keeping them 2–3cm apart, and spread lightly.

Cook for 3–4 minutes or until the surface looks dry and set and the base is lightly browned. Turn over with a spatula and cook on the other side for a further 3 minutes until lightly browned and cooked through. Keep warm while you prepare the rest of the fritters. Serve warm with fat-free natural yoghurt mixed with finely chopped fresh mint and lemon wedges for squeezing.

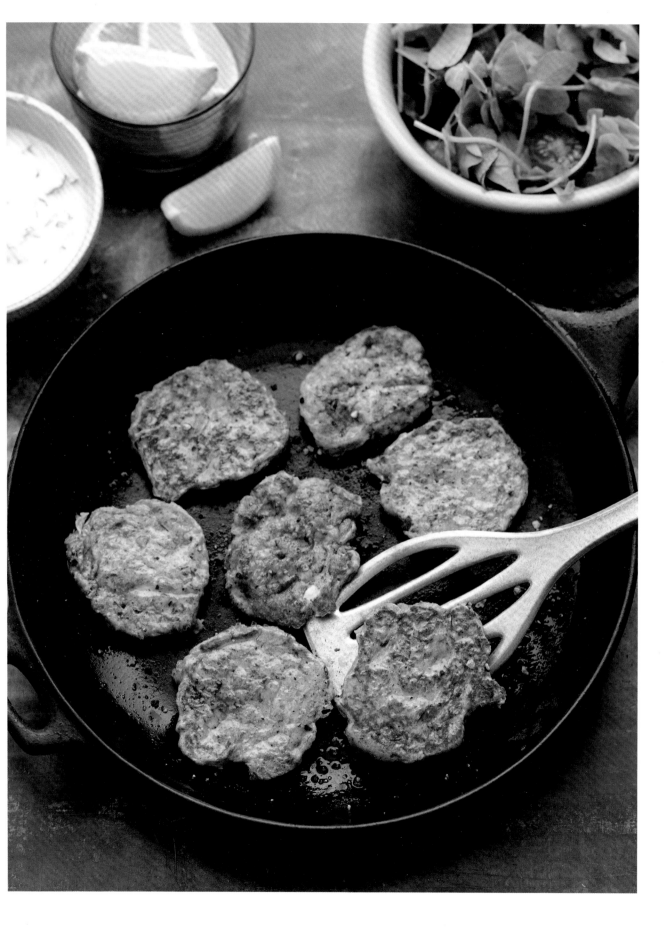

260 CALORIES PER SERVING

beany burritos

SERVES 6

PREP: 10 MINUTES

COOK: 25 MINUTES

oil, for spraying or brushing
1 medium onion, thinly
    sliced
1 yellow pepper, deseeded
    and thinly sliced
1 tsp hot smoked paprika
400g can chopped
    tomatoes with herbs
2 tbsp tomato purée
400g can red kidney beans,
    drained and rinsed
50g sliced jalapeños (from
    a jar) drained and roughly
    chopped
20g fresh coriander, leaves
    roughly chopped
6 regular flour tortilla wraps
    (each about 60g)
60g ready-grated
    mozzarella
lime wedges, to serve
    (optional)
ground black pepper

Freeze the cooled,
assembled burritos by
wrapping tightly in foil
and placing in a labelled
zip-seal bag. Freeze for
up to 1 month. Unwrap and
reheat on a baking tray from
frozen in a preheated oven
at 200°C/Fan 180°C/Gas 6
for around 10 minutes or
until lightly browned and
hot throughout.

These folded wraps are filled with a spicy combination of canned beans and tomatoes with grated cheese. They can be warmed up in the microwave if you need to make them ahead of time – perfect for a working lunch.

Spray or brush a medium non-stick saucepan with oil. Add the onion and pepper and fry gently for 3–4 minutes until lightly browned. Stir in the paprika and cook for a few seconds more.

Tip the tomatoes into the pan and add the tomato purée and beans. Bring to a gentle simmer, then cover loosely with a lid and cook for 20 minutes, stirring occasionally until thick. Take the pan off the heat and season with black pepper, then stir in the jalapeños and coriander.

Warm the tortillas for a few seconds in the microwave or a few minutes in a low oven, according to packet instructions, to make them easier to fold.

To assemble, spoon a sixth of the hot bean mixture onto the bottom half of a tortilla, leaving a border of around 4cm. Sprinkle with cheese, add a squeeze of lime if you like, and fold up the end to cover the filling. Fold the sides in and roll to enclose the filling. Serve warm.

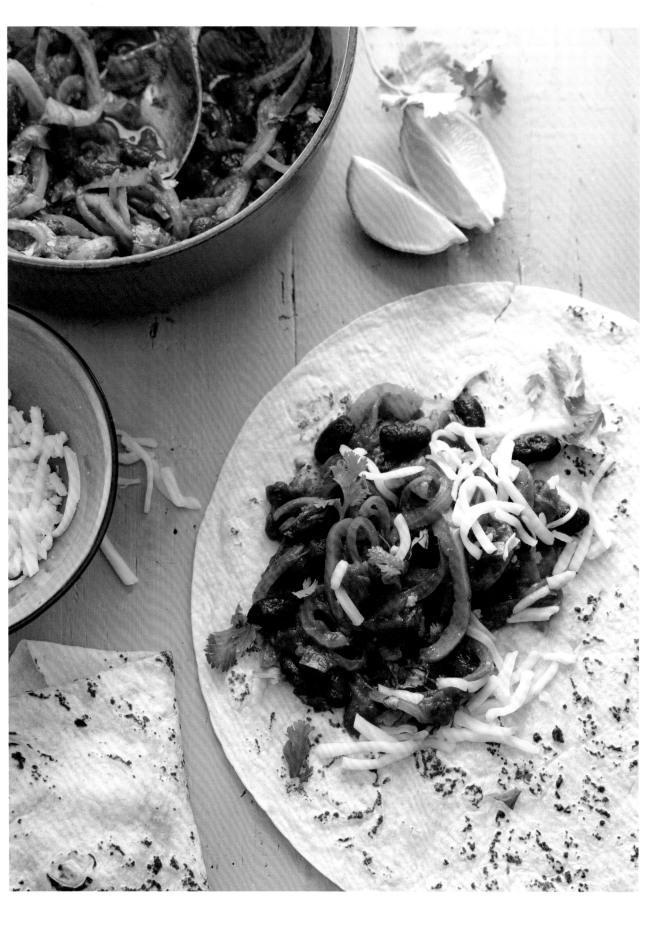

130
CALORIES
PER SERVING

pear, blue cheese and walnut salad

SERVES 4

PREP: 10 MINUTES

80g bag mixed salad leaves
1 little gem lettuce,
    leaves separated
2 firm but ripe pears,
    quartered, cored
    and sliced
25g shelled walnuts
    or pecan nuts
50g tangy blue cheese,
    such as Roquefort
    or St Agur

**FOR THE BLUE
CHEESE DRESSING**
3 tbsp fat-free natural
    yoghurt
½ tsp white wine vinegar
10g strong blue cheese such
    as Roquefort or St Agur
flaked sea salt
freshly ground black pepper

A fresh-tasting fruity salad that makes a simple lunch for four or a starter for six. I put some of the blue cheese into the dressing as well as on top as it means I get all the tangy, salty flavour through the leaves without needing to use too much cheese. Using a tangy blue cheese rather than a very creamy one means it will go further too.

To make the dressing, mix together the yoghurt and vinegar until well combined. Crumble the cheese into the dressing, season with a little salt and black pepper and mix together.

Shake the salad leaves onto a platter, top with the pears and break the blue cheese into small chunks on top. Break the nuts into pieces with your fingers and scatter them over. Serve immediately.

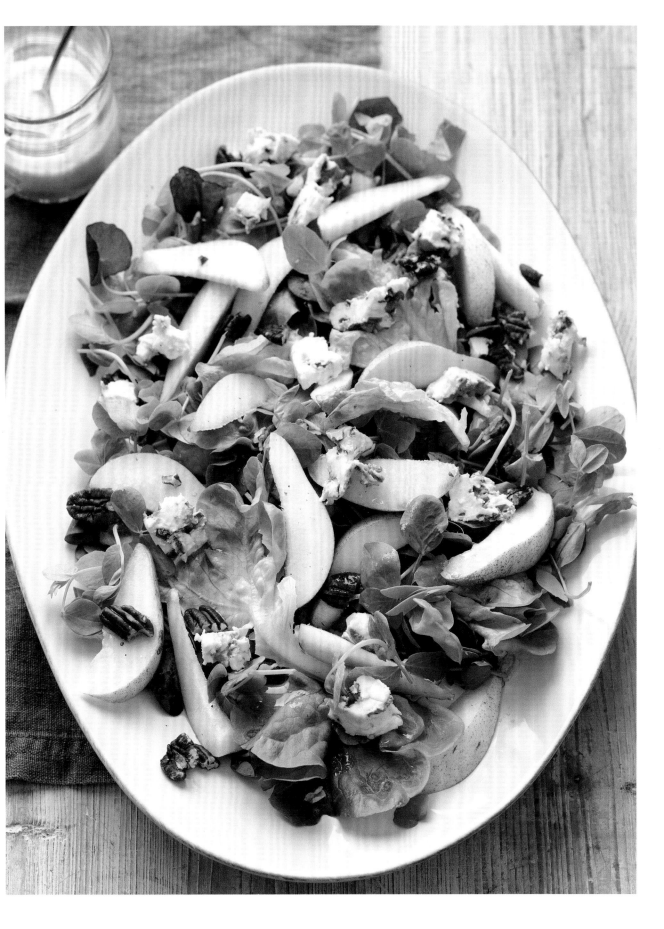

251

CALORIES
PER SERVING

egg fried rice

SERVES 3

PREP: 10 MINUTES

COOK: 10 MINUTES

3 tsp sunflower oil
2 eggs, beaten
1 red and 1 yellow pepper,
    deseeded and thinly
    sliced
150g button mushrooms,
    wiped and sliced
50g frozen peas
6 spring onions, trimmed
    and sliced
250g pouch cooked
    long-grain rice
dark soy sauce, to serve

A filling dish that can be served alongside other Chinese-style dishes and simple grilled meat or fish, but equally good served just as it is, in deep bowls, for a hearty weekend lunch or fuss-free supper. As an accompaniment for four, each serving contains 189 calories.

Heat a teaspoon of the oil in a large non-stick frying pan or wok. Add the beaten eggs and swirl around the pan to make a thin omelette. Cook over a medium-high heat for 1 minute or until almost set, then break into rough strips with a wooden spoon and transfer to a plate.

Return the pan to the heat and add the remaining oil. Stir-fry the peppers and mushrooms for 3 minutes. Add the peas, spring onions and rice and cook for a further 3 minutes or until hot, while stirring.

Return the egg to the pan and stir through the rice and vegetables for 1 minute or until steaming and hot, stirring continuously. Serve with soy sauce.

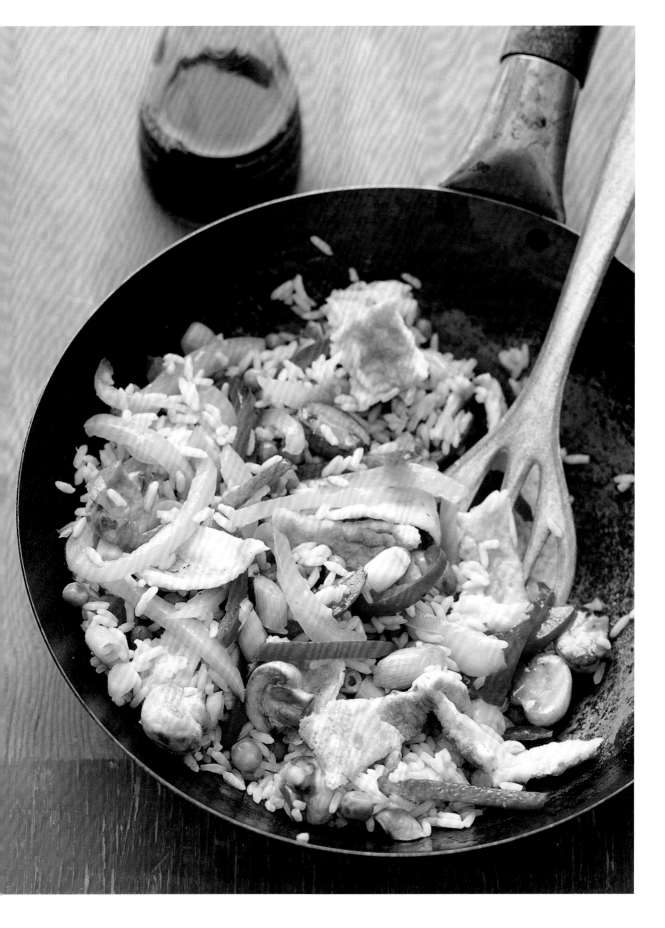

313
CALORIES
PER SERVING

curried courgette omelette

SERVES 1

PREP: 5 MINUTES

COOK: 6 MINUTES

1 medium courgette
   (about 225g)
2 eggs
1/2 tsp medium curry powder
oil, for spraying or brushing
25g feta cheese, drained
8 cherry tomatoes, halved
flaked sea salt
freshly ground black pepper

Tip: This omelette is great
filled with rocket and baby
spinach leaves just before
folding.

Use a really good non-stick flameproof pan with a base
of around 20cm in diameter for this recipe. Adding grated
courgette to the eggs will make the omelette more filling and
the hint of curry powder brings a welcome touch of spice.

Coarsely grate the courgette, then squeeze handfuls over
the sink to extract as much liquid as possible.

Beat the eggs with a large metal whisk until smooth, then
thoroughly whisk in the curry powder. Season with a little
salt and some freshly ground black pepper. Stir in the grated
courgette. Preheat the grill to its hottest setting.

Spray or brush a medium non-stick flameproof frying pan
with oil and place over a medium heat. Pour the egg mixture
into the frying pan and cook for 3 minutes or until the bottom
is golden brown. Scatter the feta and tomatoes over the
omelette and place the pan under the hot grill. Cook for
a further 2–3 minutes or until the eggs are just set. (Make
sure you don't put the handle under the grill.)

Remove the pan from the heat, carefully loosen the sides of
the omelette with a heatproof palette knife and slide it onto
a warmed plate, folding it as you do so. Serve with a large,
lightly dressed salad.

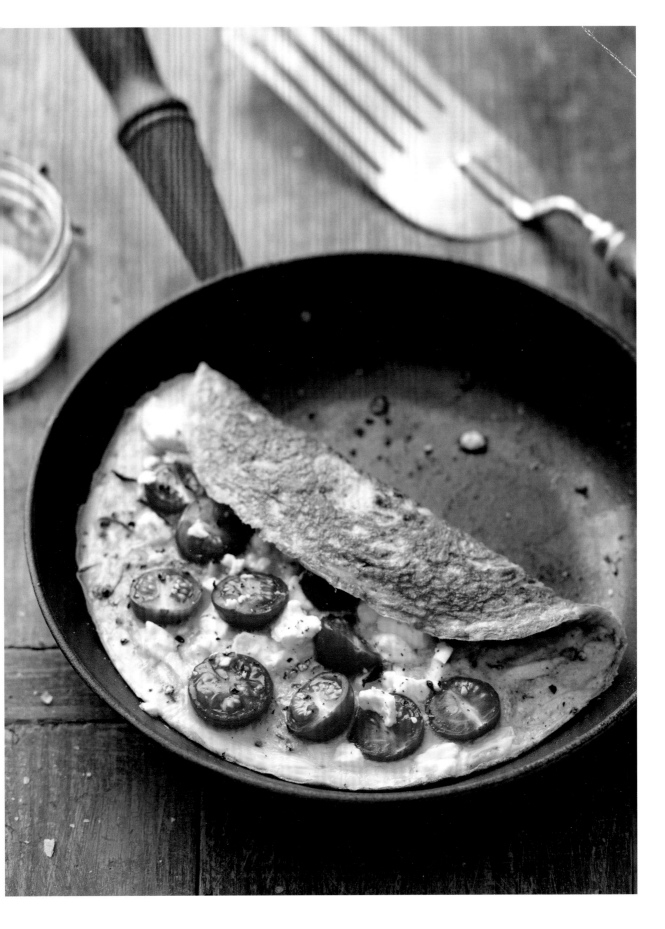

246
CALORIES
PER SERVING

moroccan chickpea stew

SERVES 4

PREP: 10 MINUTES

COOK: 25 MINUTES

1 tbsp sunflower oil
2 medium onions, thinly
 sliced
4 garlic cloves, crushed
25g chunk fresh root ginger,
 peeled and finely grated
1 tsp cumin seeds
1 tbsp ground coriander
2 tbsp harissa paste
400g can chopped
 tomatoes
2 x 400g cans chickpeas,
 drained and rinsed
2 tbsp tomato purée
1 tbsp clear honey
½ tsp flaked sea salt,
 plus extra to season
good pinch of saffron
1 tsp caster sugar
350ml vegetable stock
 (made with 1 vegetable
 stock cube)
15g fresh coriander, leaves
 roughly chopped, plus
 extra leaves to garnish
1–2 tbsp fresh lemon juice,
 to taste
ground black pepper

Freeze the cooled stew in
a freezer-proof container
for up to 2 months. Defrost
overnight in the fridge.
Reheat in a large non-stick
saucepan over a medium
heat, stirring regularly until
piping hot throughout.

**This stew uses canned chickpeas to save time and is
flavoured with warming ginger, spices and chilli. I sometimes
stir cubed sweet potato or butternut squash into the stew
along with the chickpeas to make more of a one pot meal.
Serve with spoonfuls of fat-free natural yoghurt and freshly
cooked vegetables or salad.**

Heat the oil in a large wide-based saucepan or non-stick
sauté pan. Add the onions and fry over a medium heat
for 5 minutes, stirring occasionally until softened and
lightly browned.

Stir in the garlic, ginger, cumin seeds, ground coriander
and harissa. Tip the tomatoes and chickpeas into the pan
and stir in the tomato purée, honey, salt, saffron, sugar
and stock.

Bring to the boil then reduce the heat, so the sauce simmers
gently and cook for about 20 minutes, stirring regularly until
the sauce is thick. If the sauce becomes too thick before the
time is up, add a little water.

Stir in the chopped coriander then season with salt and pepper
and add the lemon juice to taste. Garnish with more coriander
leaves just before serving.

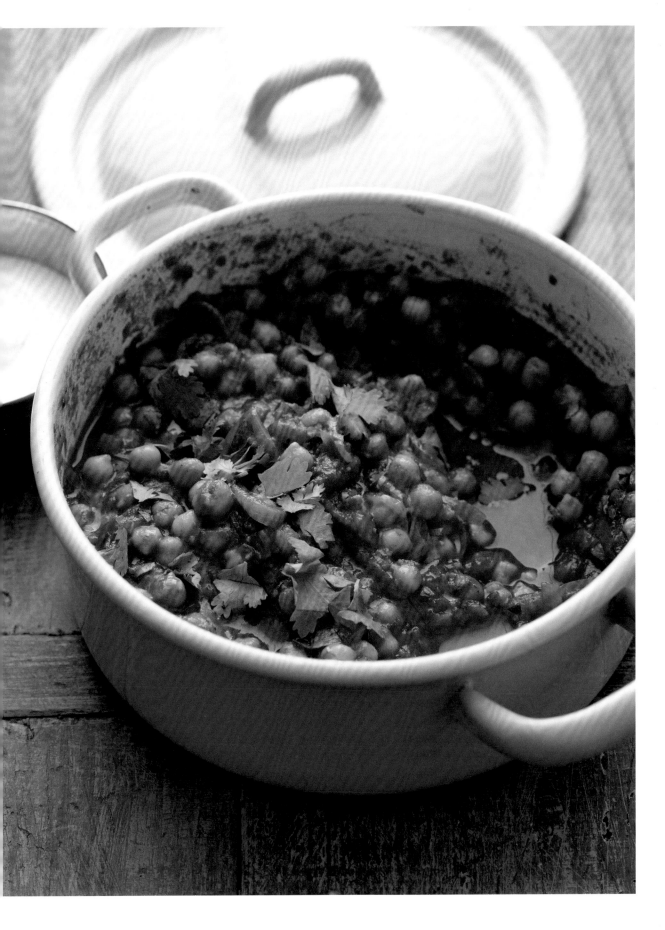

364

warm vegetable, goat's cheese and lentil salad

SERVES 4
PREP: 10 MINUTES
COOK: 10 MINUTES

450g sweet potatoes, peeled and cut into roughly 2cm chunks
1 red pepper, deseeded and cut into 2cm chunks
2 medium courgettes, cut into roughly 1cm slices
1 red onion, cut into 6 wedges
1 tbsp sunflower or mild olive oil
250g sachet ready-to-eat puy lentils
2 tbsp thick balsamic vinegar
1 tsp extra virgin olive oil
150g soft, rindless goat's cheese
fresh mint or basil leaves, to garnish
flaked sea salt
ground black pepper
tomato dressing (see right), to serve

Sachets of ready-to-eat lentils make a handy low-fat addition to any meal. They work particularly well in this warm salad of pan-fried vegetables and goat's cheese. If you can't find pre-cooked lentils, cook 125g dried puy lentils instead. Drizzle with a fresh tomato dressing (see below) or balsamic vinegar.

Half fill a medium saucepan with water, add the sweet potato and bring to the boil. Cook for 5 minutes or until just tender then drain well.

Put all the raw vegetables in a bowl, add the sweet potatoes and toss with the sunflower oil. Season with a pinch of salt and ground black pepper.

Place a large non-stick frying pan or wok over a high heat and stir-fry the vegetables for 5 minutes or until lightly browned. Tip into a warmed heat-proof bowl. Add the puy lentils to the pan and stir fry for 2–3 minutes more or until hot, then stir into the vegetables.

Stir the balsamic vinegar and oil through the lentils and vegetables. Divide between four plates and break the goat's cheese on top. Garnish with mint or basil leaves and serve.

Tomato dressing: Cut 2 large ripe tomatoes in half and remove the seeds. Roughly chop the tomatoes and place in a jug with ½ small garlic clove, 1 teaspoon thick balsamic vinegar and 2 teaspoons extra virgin olive oil. Blitz with a stick blender until as smooth as possible. Season with a little salt and pepper and toss with the lentil salad. Serves 4. Calories per serving: 27

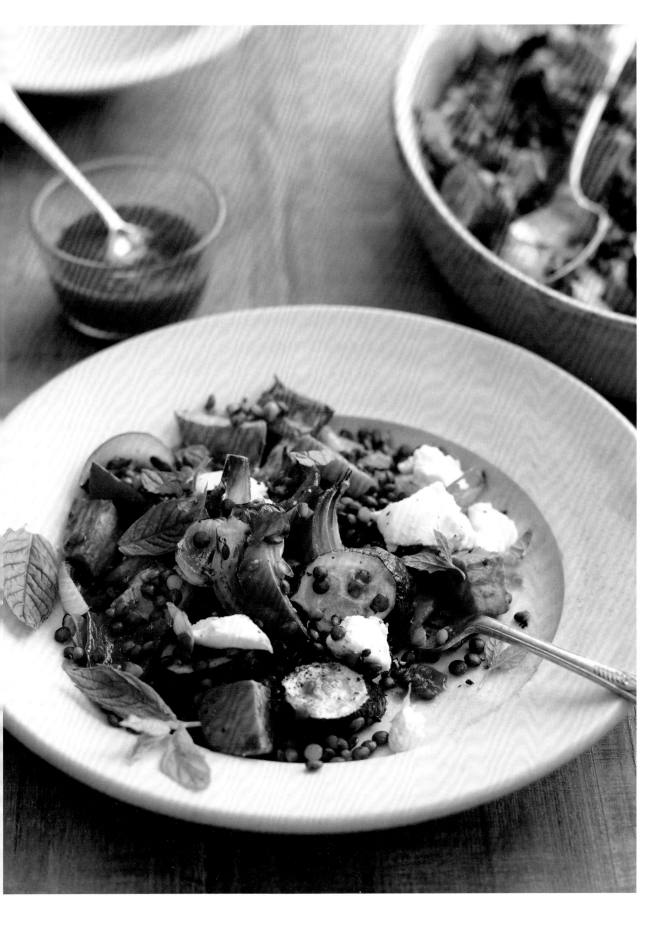

ratatouille

This simple ratatouille is made with chunky vegetables in a rich, garlicky tomato sauce. I like to serve it at room temperature, tossed with a few fresh basil leaves. Perfect with grilled or barbecued meats and fish or on its own for a super-low-calorie meal.

SERVES 4
PREP: 10 MINUTES
COOK: 30 MINUTES

2 medium courgettes, halved lengthways and cut into roughly 2cm chunks
2 mixed colour peppers, deseeded and cut roughly into 3cm chunks
1 medium aubergine, cut into roughly 2.5cm chunks
1 large onion, cut into thin wedges
1 tbsp sunflower oil
½ tsp fine sea salt, plus extra to season
4 garlic cloves, thinly sliced
1 tsp coriander seeds, lightly crushed
400g can chopped tomatoes
2 tbsp tomato purée
handful fresh basil leaves, roughly torn
1 tbsp extra virgin olive oil, to serve (optional)
freshly ground black pepper

Freeze the ratatouille in shallow freezer-proof containers, without adding the basil leaves, for up to 2 months. Defrost overnight in the fridge. Tip into a large saucepan and reheat thoroughly. Toss with fresh basil leaves before serving.

Put the courgettes, peppers, aubergine and onion in a large bowl. Pour over the sunflower oil and season with salt and lots of ground black pepper. Toss well together.

Place a large, deep non-stick frying pan or sauté pan over a high heat and stir-fry the vegetables in two batches for 3–4 minutes until lightly browned, putting the first batch on a plate while you cook the second batch.

Add the garlic and coriander seeds and cook for 1 minute before returning the first batch of vegetables to the pan. Add the tomatoes and bring to a simmer. Reduce the heat and cook the ratatouille at a gentle simmer for 20 minutes, stirring occasionally. It is done when the vegetables are softened and the sauce is thick.

Season with a little salt if needed and plenty of ground black pepper. Eat warm or cold, tossed with a few torn basil leaves. Drizzle with extra virgin olive oil just before serving if you like, but remember to add an extra 99 calories for each tablespoon.

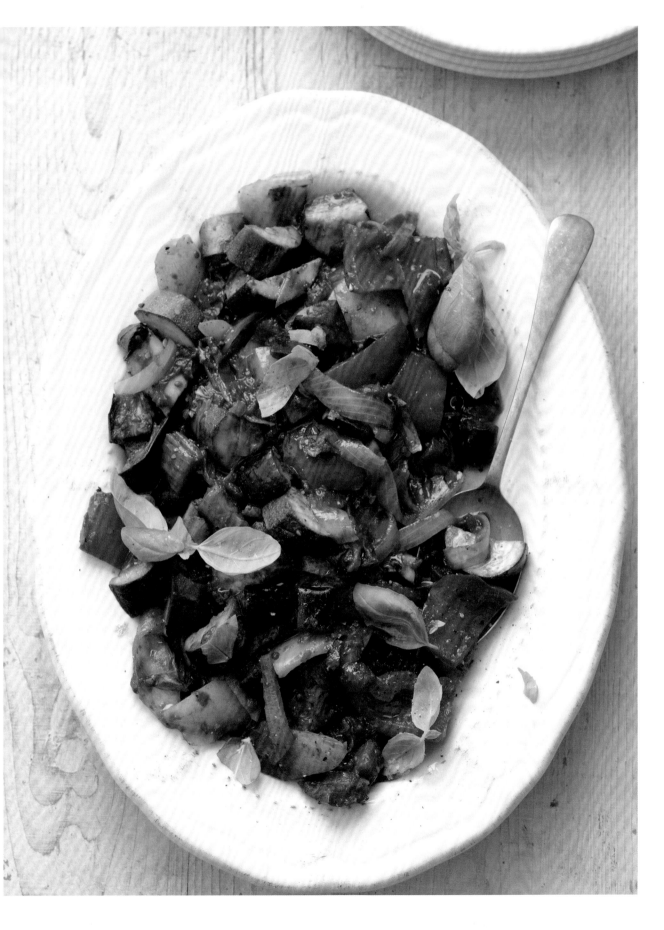

192 CALORIES
PER SERVING

english garden egg salad

SERVES 4

PREP: 5 MINUTES

COOK: 10 MINUTES

4 large fridge-cold eggs
3 little gem lettuces,
    leaves separated
4 ripe tomatoes, quartered
⅓ cucumber (about 100g),
    halved lengthways
    and sliced
1 large carrot, peeled
    and coarsely grated
2 celery sticks, sliced
100g radishes, halved or
    quartered if large
fresh salad cress, for
    snipping

FOR THE DRESSING
3 tbsp salad cream
1 tbsp cold water

This might not be the most exciting salad, but it's one that I go back to again and again. I tend to use whatever I have in my fridge and often add sliced ham too, which is roughly 32 calories for a regular slice.

Half fill a small saucepan with water and bring to the boil. Gently add the eggs to the water and return to the boil. (If you add the eggs too quickly or roughly, the shells could crack.)

Cook the eggs for 9 minutes. Drain and immerse in cold water until cool enough to handle. Peel off the shells and cut the eggs into quarters.

Wash and drain the lettuce leaves and put into a large bowl. Add the tomatoes, cucumber, pepper, celery and radishes. Toss lightly and snip fresh cress over the top.

To make the dressing, mix the salad cream with the water until smooth. Drizzle over the salad to serve.

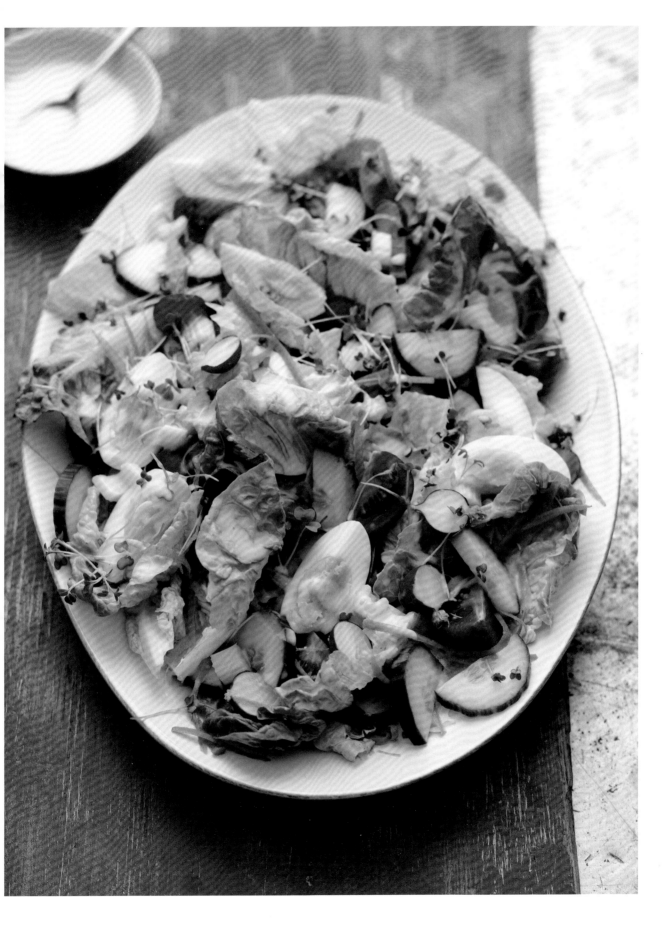

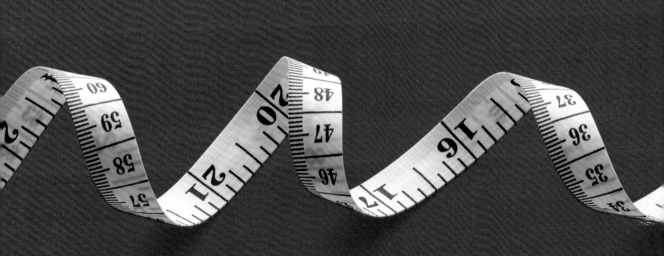

soups
and snacks

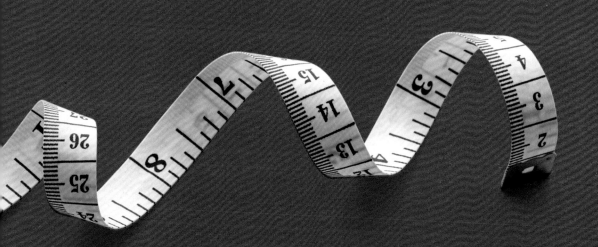

111
CALORIES
PER SERVING

cooling cucumber and avocado soup

SERVES 4

PREP: 5 MINUTES

½ large cucumber, peeled
1 firm but ripe medium
    avocado
1 garlic clove, chopped
10g fresh mint, leaves
    finely chopped
1 heaped tbsp roughly
    chopped fresh chives
150g fat-free natural
    yoghurt
100ml semi-skimmed milk,
    well chilled
flaked sea salt
ground black pepper

Flat freeze the soup in
labelled zip-seal bags.
Defrost overnight in
the fridge and stir well
before serving.

A cooling summer soup that makes a refreshing summer lunch, served with slices of warm ciabatta. Try adding a couple of ice cubes to each bowl if the weather is particularly warm.

Cut the cucumber into short lengths and put in a food processor or blender. Cut the avocado in half and remove the stone. Scoop out the flesh with a large spoon and add to the cucumber.

Drop the garlic, mint and chives on top. Add the yoghurt and milk, a good pinch of salt and lots of ground black pepper. Blitz until as smooth as possible. Adjust seasoning to taste.

Serve in small bowls with warm bread or breadsticks.

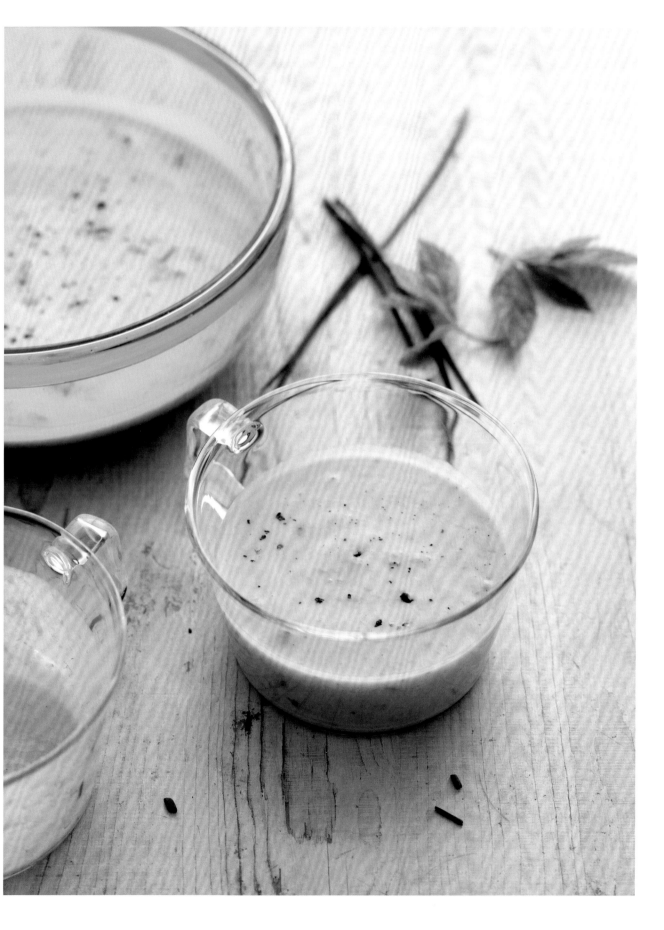

67 CALORIES PER SERVING

throw-it-together vegetable soup

SERVES 6

PREP: 15 MINUTES

COOK: 20 MINUTES

2 tsp olive oil
1 medium onion,
 finely chopped
2 garlic cloves, thinly sliced
2 sticks celery, thinly sliced
2 carrots, peeled and cut
 into roughly 1.5cm dice
400g can chopped
 tomatoes with herbs
2 tbsp tomato purée
2 chicken or vegetable
 stock cubes
1.5 litres water
2 courgettes, cut into
 2cm chunks
150g green beans, cut
 into roughly 2cm lengths
100g frozen peas
flaked sea salt
ground black pepper

Freeze the cooled soup
in freezer-proof containers.
Cover tightly and freeze
for up to 3 months. To serve,
warm through gently in
a large saucepan until
thawed, then simmer until
piping hot, stirring regularly.

A dieter's best friend, this filling soup is simple to put together and keeps well in the fridge for up to 3 days. Dip into a bowl when you are feeling peckish and you'll find it much easier to keep the lid firmly on the biscuit tin.

Heat the oil in a large non-stick saucepan and fry the onion, garlic, celery and carrots gently for 5 minutes, stirring often.

Add the chopped tomatoes and tomato purée, crumble over the stock cubes and stir in the water. Bring to the boil, then reduce the heat slightly and cook for 5 minutes, stirring occasionally.

Add the courgettes, green beans and peas and simmer for a further 5 minutes or until the vegetables are just tender. Season the soup with a little salt if needed and lots of black pepper. Serve in warm, deep bowls.

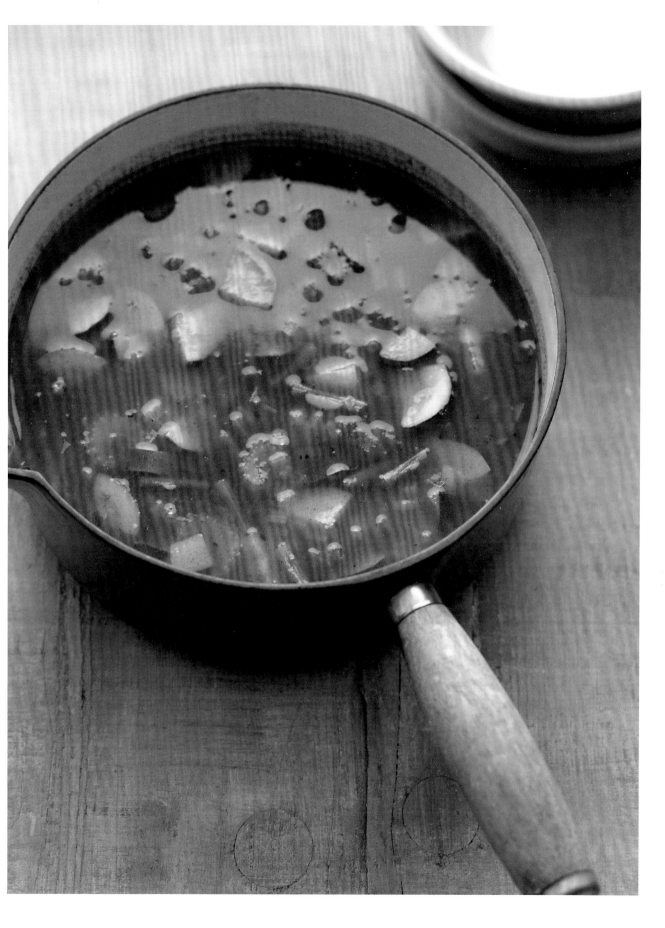

89
CALORIES
PER SERVING

tom yum soup

SERVES 4

PREP: 10–15 MINUTES

COOK: 5 MINUTES

500ml fresh chicken stock
500ml cold water
2 tbsp tom yum paste
1–2 tbsp Thai fish sauce
 (nam pla)
1 long red chilli, thinly sliced
175g raw, peeled king
 prawns, thawed if frozen
100g baby corn, halved
 lengthways
100g mangetout, trimmed
5 fresh, frozen or dried
 Kaffir lime leaves
 (optional)
juice of ½ lime
15g fresh coriander leaves

This soothing soup can be knocked together with very few ingredients. Tom yum paste is now widely available in supermarkets as well as Asian stores. I like to chuck in a few Kaffir lime leaves – either fresh or frozen – and you can use fresh or frozen coriander too.

Pour the stock and water into a large saucepan and bring to the boil. Stir in the tom yum paste, a tablespoon of the fish sauce and the sliced chilli. Reduce the heat to a simmer.

Add the prawns, baby corn, mangetout and lime leaves, if using, to the soup and simmer gently for 2–3 minutes or until the prawns are pink and hot throughout.

Stir in the lime juice and add a little more fish sauce if needed. The soup should have a spicy, hot and sour flavour. Ladle the soup into four large, deep bowls and sprinkle with the coriander.

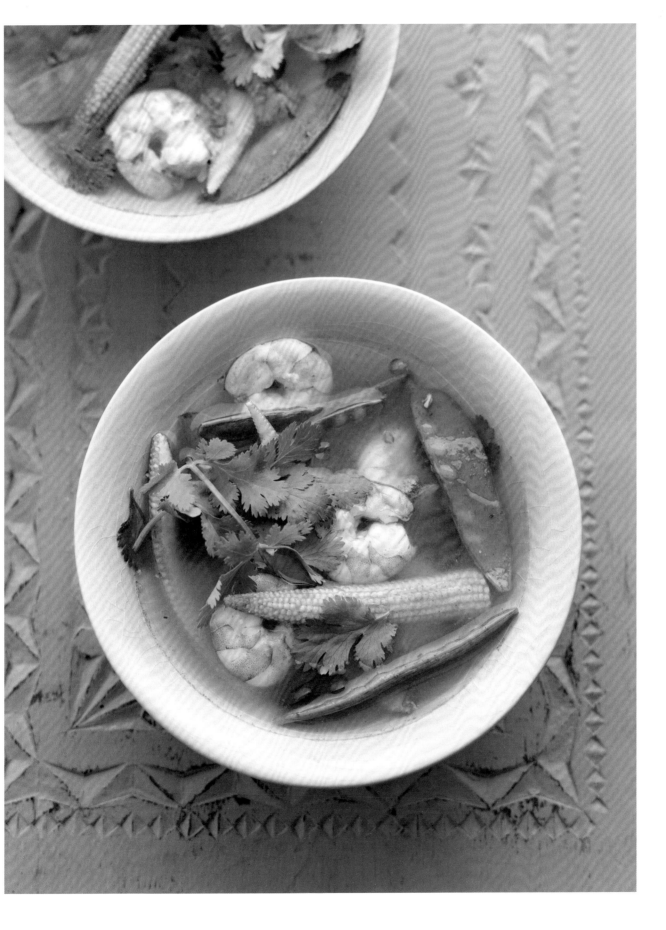

89 CALORIES PER SERVING

minted pea soup

SERVES 4
PREP: 5 MINUTES
COOK: 10 MINUTES

1 small onion, roughly
    chopped
2 garlic cloves, roughly
    chopped
500g frozen peas
750ml vegetable or
    chicken stock (made
    with 1 stock cube)
½ tsp dried mint
flaked sea salt
ground black pepper

Flat freeze the cooled soup
in freezer bags. To serve,
warm through gently in a
large saucepan until thawed
then simmer until piping
hot, stirring regularly.

A delicious soup made from ingredients that you probably
have knocking around the kitchen. Perfect for a light lunch or
supper. Save calories by serving with plain breadsticks instead
of toast; they are only around 25 calories each.

Place the onion, garlic, peas and stock in a medium saucepan
and bring to a simmer. Cook for 5 minutes, stirring occasionally.

Remove the pan from the heat, stir in the mint and blitz with
a stick blender until smooth. Or leave to cool for a few minutes
and blend in a food processor. Pass through a sieve for an
extra smooth soup.

Season with salt and pepper and serve.

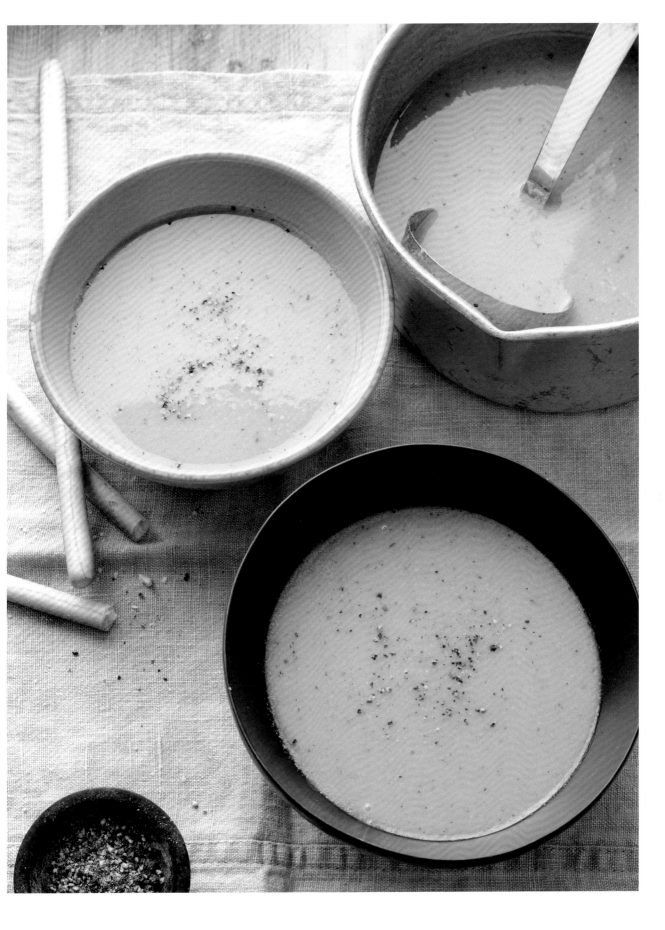

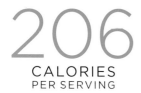

206
CALORIES
PER SERVING

poppadum toppers

1 large ripe tomato,
   roughly chopped
¼ small red onion,
   finely chopped
½ tsp thick balsamic
   vinegar
small handful fresh basil
   leaves, shredded
½ firm but ripe avocado
2 ready-to-eat poppadums,
   from a packet
1 skinless cooked chicken
   breast (about 100g),
   sliced
flaked sea salt
ground black pepper

Ready-to-eat poppadums contain around 35 calories each and make a crunchy addition to a quick snack. Break into pieces and use to scoop up lean chicken, avocado and fresh tomato salsa.

Mix the tomato, onion, balsamic vinegar and basil leaves together lightly to make a salsa. Season with salt and ground black pepper.

Cut the avocado in half and remove the stone. Use a large serving spoon to scoop out the flesh and put it on a board. Cut it into slices.

Divide the poppadums between two plates and serve with the sliced chicken, avocado and tomato and basil salsa.

Egg with ham and cress: Divide 50g wafer-thin slices of smoked ham and 1 halved hard-boiled egg between two plates. Scatter with freshly snipped cress if you like and serve with 2 ready-to-eat poppadums. Serves 2. Calories per serving: 115

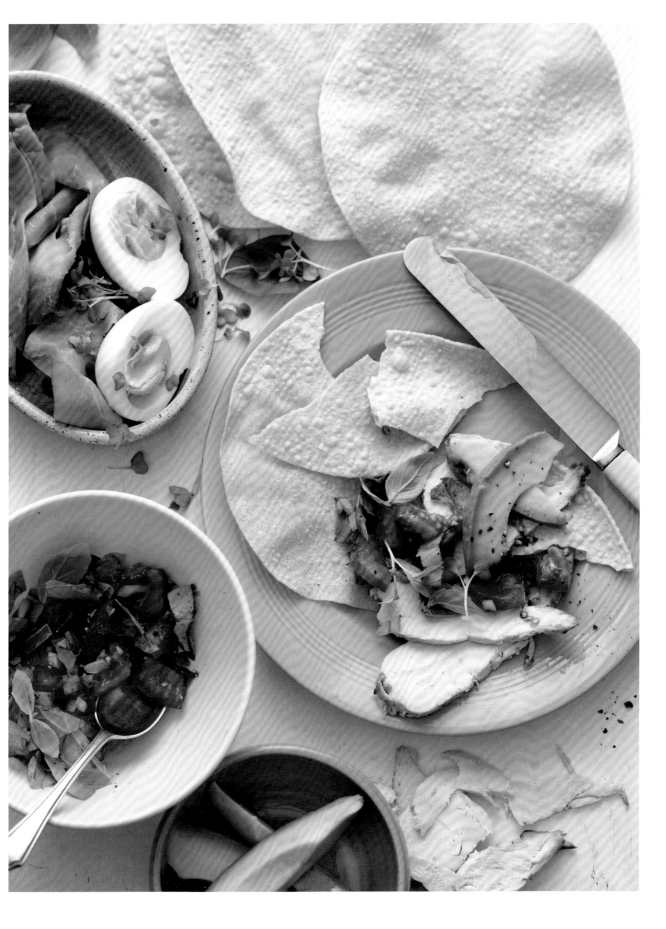

142
CALORIES
PER SERVING

smoked trout pâté pot

SERVES 4
PREP: 10 MINUTES

200g skinless smoked
   trout fillets
½ small onion
100g quark (naturally
   fat-free soft cheese)
2 tbsp half-fat crème fraiche
finely grated zest of
   ½ unwaxed lemon
flaked sea salt
ground black pepper
12 french bread toasts
   (see right)

TO SERVE
little gem lettuce leaves
cucumber, thinly sliced

When a bar of chocolate beckons, these little pots help prevent me succumbing. They make a great light lunch and can be taken to work as long as you keep them cold. Make a big batch of French bread toasts and serve a couple as I've done here.

Flake the trout into a food processor. Peel the onion and coarsely grate it onto a board. Hold the grated onion and squeeze it hard over the trout to release the juice – this will add flavour to the pâté. Discard the onion flesh.

Add the quark, crème fraiche and lemon zest to the trout and season well with a good pinch of salt and plenty of ground black pepper.

Blitz all the ingredients together until as smooth as possible. Adjust the seasoning to taste and add a little more lemon juice if needed. Spoon the mixture into four glass tumblers or small rubber-sealed jars with lettuce leaves and sliced cucumber.

Avocado and prawn pot: Cut 1 firm but ripe medium avocado in half and remove the stone. Use a large serving spoon to scoop out the flesh and put on a board. Cut into slices and toss with 1 tablespoon of fresh lemon juice. Mix 2 tablespoons light mayonnaise, 2 tablespoons fat-free natural yoghurt, 1 tablespoon tomato ketchup and a small splash Worcestershire sauce. Season to taste. Stir 100g cooked and peeled prawns (thawed if frozen) into the mayonnaise. Spoon the mixture into four glass tumblers or small rubber-sealed jars with the avocado, shredded lettuce leaves and sliced tomatoes. Serves 4. Calories per serving: 124

French bread toasts: Slice a baton loaf (short sandwich baguette) diagonally and very thinly (around 5g per slice). Place the slices on a baking sheet and dry in a preheated oven at 180°C/ Fan 160°C/Gas 4 for about 15 minutes. Leave to cool. Store in a sealed container. Eat within 7 days or freeze. Warm through before serving if you like. Makes 25 slices. Calories per slice: 13

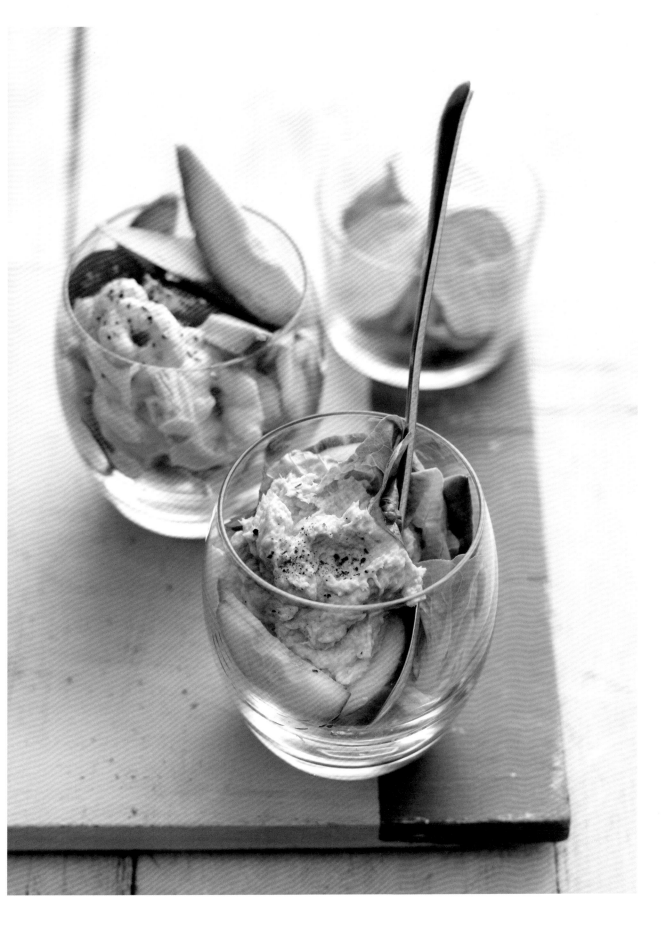

112 CALORIES PER SERVING

frittata bites

SERVES 6
PREP: 10 MINUTES
COOK: 20 MINUTES

1 tbsp olive oil
1 medium onion, finely
    chopped
1 garlic clove, crushed
1 red and 1 yellow pepper,
    deseeded and diced into
    roughly 1cm cubes
25g hard chorizo, skinned
    and very finely diced
4 eggs, beaten
1 tsp flaked sea salt
freshly ground black pepper

Freeze the bites in a rigid
freezer-proof container,
interleaved with baking
parchment. Defrost in the
fridge overnight and serve
cold or heat from frozen,
4–6 at a time, on a plate
in the microwave for about
1½ minutes on its highest
setting until hot throughout.

Baked in a mini muffin tin, these frittata bites pack a powerful flavour punch and are just the thing to take the edge off your appetite between meals. My muffin tin has 24 holes but if you have a smaller one, simply make the bites in separate batches. Each bite contains 28 calories.

Heat the oil in a non-stick frying pan. Add the onion and cook for 3 minutes over a medium heat until beginning to colour, stirring occasionally. Preheat the oven to 200°C/Fan 180°C/Gas 6.

Add the garlic, peppers and chorizo to the frying pan, season well with salt and plenty of freshly ground black pepper and cook for a further 3 minutes, while stirring. Divide everything between the holes of a 24-hole mini muffin tin.

Pour the beaten eggs over the vegetables and chorizo and transfer the tin to the oven. Bake for 10 minutes or until slightly risen, firm and golden.

Take out of the oven and turn the frittata bites out onto a board. Serve warm or leave to cool then pack into a rigid container, cover and keep in the fridge for up to 2 days.

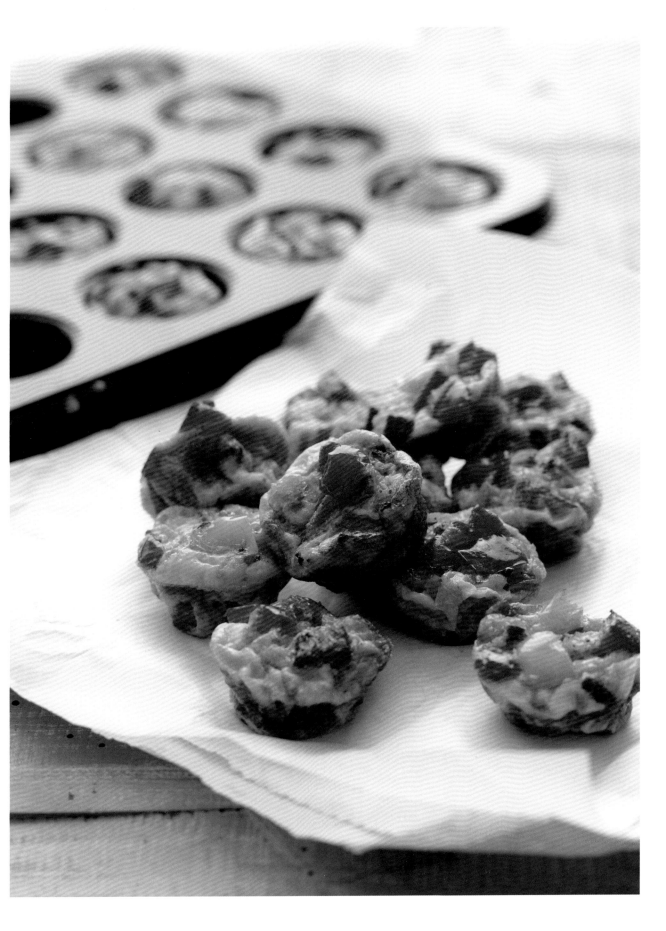

99
CALORIES
PER SERVING

chicken tikka strips

SERVES 4

**PREP: 5 MINUTES,
PLUS MARINATING TIME**

COOK: 6–10 MINUTES

325g chicken breast
   mini fillets
1 tbsp tikka curry paste
4 tbsp fat-free natural
   yoghurt
flaked sea salt
ground black pepper

Lean chicken breast makes a convenient, low-fat snack and when it's been marinated, it's extra delicious. I use chicken mini fillets for this recipe, but you could cut skinless boneless chicken breasts into thin strips too. Serve just as they are or scatter onto salads or use to top open sandwiches. If you don't have time to marinate the chicken, just coat well in the spice or herb mix and grill straight away.

Put the chicken mini fillets in a bowl and stir in the tikka paste, yoghurt, a pinch of salt and a good grind of black pepper. Cover and leave to marinate in the fridge for up to 1 hour.

Arrange the chicken pieces on a rack over a grill pan lined with foil. Cook the fillets under a preheated hot grill for 6–10 minutes without turning, until lightly browned and cooked through. (There should be no pinkness remaining in the centre of the chicken when it is cut.)

Sun-dried tomato pesto strips: Put the chicken fillets in a bowl and stir in 2 tablespoons sun-dried tomato pesto and a good grind of black pepper. Cover and leave to marinate in the fridge for up to 1 hour. Cook as above. Serves 4. Calories per serving: 110

Lemon and coriander strips: Put the chicken fillets in a bowl and stir in 3 tablespoons fresh lemon juice, 2 tablespoons finely chopped fresh coriander and ½ teaspoon ground coriander, a pinch of salt and a good grind of black pepper. Cook as above. Serves 4. Calories per serving: 87

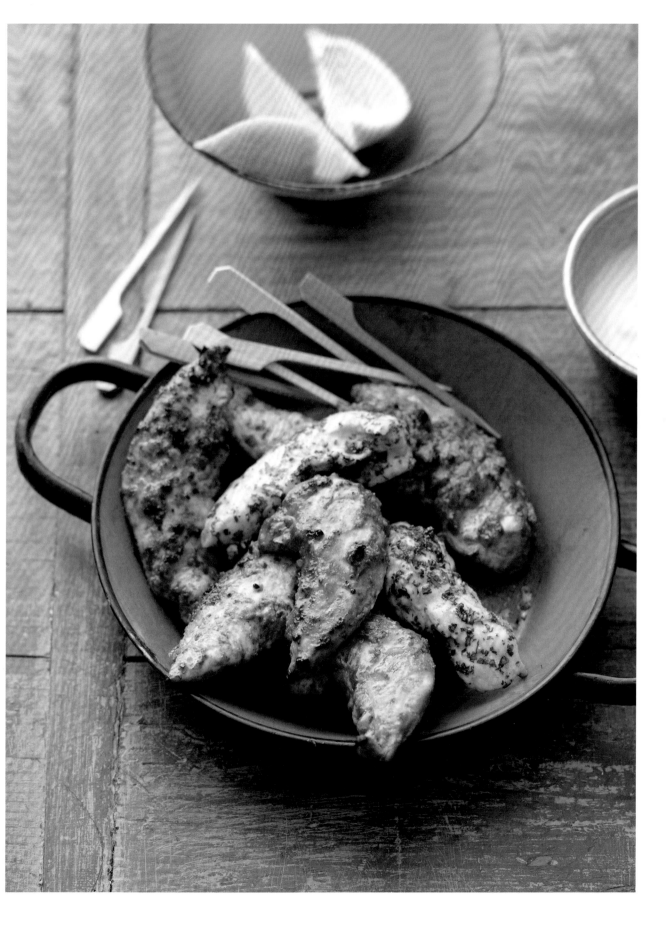

42
CALORIES
PER SERVING

harissa hummus

SERVES 6

PREP: 5 MINUTES

100g hummus
100g fat-free fromage frais
2 tsp harissa paste
finely grated zest of
   ½ lemon

When time is short, it's easy to jazz up ready-made dips rather than starting from scratch. The best way to reduce calories is to add ingredients that are very low in fat, such as fat-free fromage frais. Serve with crunchy vegetable sticks or scoop up with my pitta dippers (see below).

Mix the hummus, fromage frais, harissa and lemon zest together in a bowl and transfer to small rubber-sealed jars if you like. Cover and keep chilled until ready to serve.

Creamy reduced-fat taramasalata: Mix 100g taramasalata with 100g fat-free fromage frais in a bowl. Cover and keep chilled until ready to serve. Serves 6. Calories per serving: 92

Pitta dippers: Warm 2 pitta breads then split them in half and cut them into strips. Scatter over a baking tray. Bake in a preheated oven at 200°C/Fan 180°C/Gas 6 for 15 minutes, turning once until crisp and lightly browned. Serves 6. Calories per serving: 51

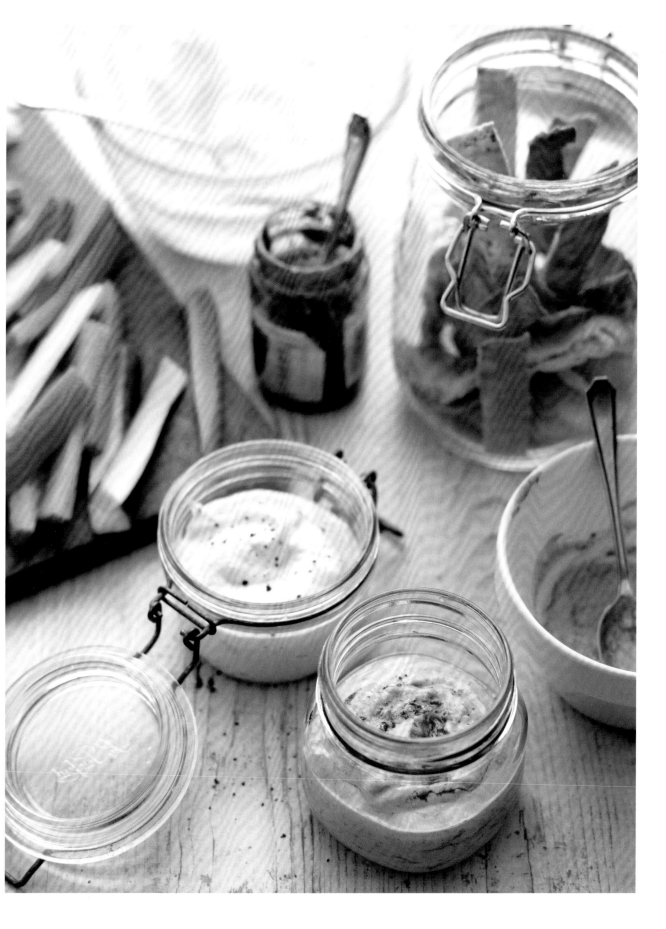

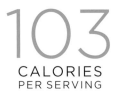

103 CALORIES PER SERVING

grilled tomatoes and cheese on toast

SERVES 4

PREP: 5 MINUTES

COOK: 5 MINUTES

4 thin slices of sourdough
   or wholemeal bread
   (each about 25g)
2 large ripe tomatoes, sliced
40g ready-grated
   mozzarella or half-fat
   Cheddar cheese
Worcestershire sauce
   (optional)
flaked sea salt
ground black pepper

Cheese on toast is one of my favourite quick lunches but it is fiendishly high in calories. This version tops the toast with slices of tomato before the cheese, so I've been able to reduce the cheese by half. Ready-grated mozzarella has roughly the same amount of calories as half-fat Cheddar and melts beautifully.

Place the bread on a rack and toast on both sides under a preheated grill. Top with the tomato slices, season with salt and pepper and return to the grill for 2–3 minutes or until the tomatoes are hot.

Scatter the cheese over the tomatoes and return to the grill until it is melted and beginning to brown. Divide the toast between four plates, add a little Worcestershire sauce if you like and serve.

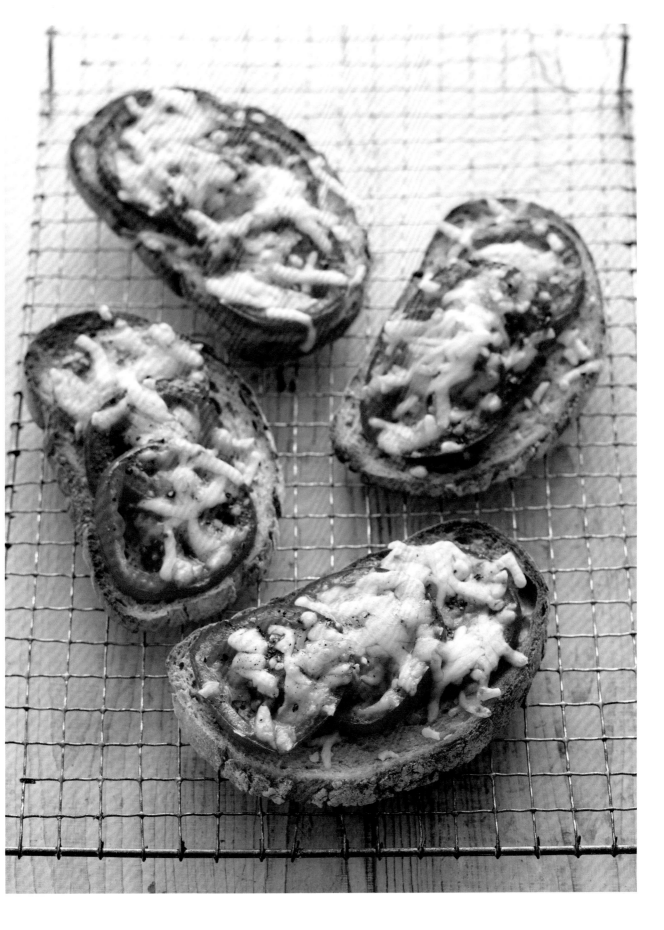

158
CALORIES
PER SERVING

salmon and cream cheese snack rolls

SERVES 1

PREP: 5 MINUTES

COOK: 2 MINUTES

1 large egg
½ tbsp finely chopped
    chives (optional)
oil, for spraying or brushing
4 tsp light soft cheese
    (such as Philadelphia),
    about 20g
20g sliced smoked salmon
flaked sea salt
ground black pepper

These low carb rolls make a simple alternative to wraps and sushi. Eat as a snack or make a few for lunch. I really like the salmon filling, but smoked ham, Parma ham and chopped hard-boiled egg make good alternatives, as do deli dips.

Break the egg into a bowl and season with salt and pepper. Beat with a metal whisk until smooth. Stir in the chives if using.

Spray or brush a small non-stick frying pan with oil and place over a medium heat. The pan should have a base no wider than 20cm.

Pour the egg into the pan and cook without stirring for 1½ minutes or until lightly browned and set. It should look like a very thin omelette. Loosen the omelette with a palette knife and transfer to a board or plate. Leave to cool for a few minutes.

Spread the omelette with the cheese and top half of it with slices of smoked salmon. Roll up from the smoked salmon side. Cut into thick slices and serve.

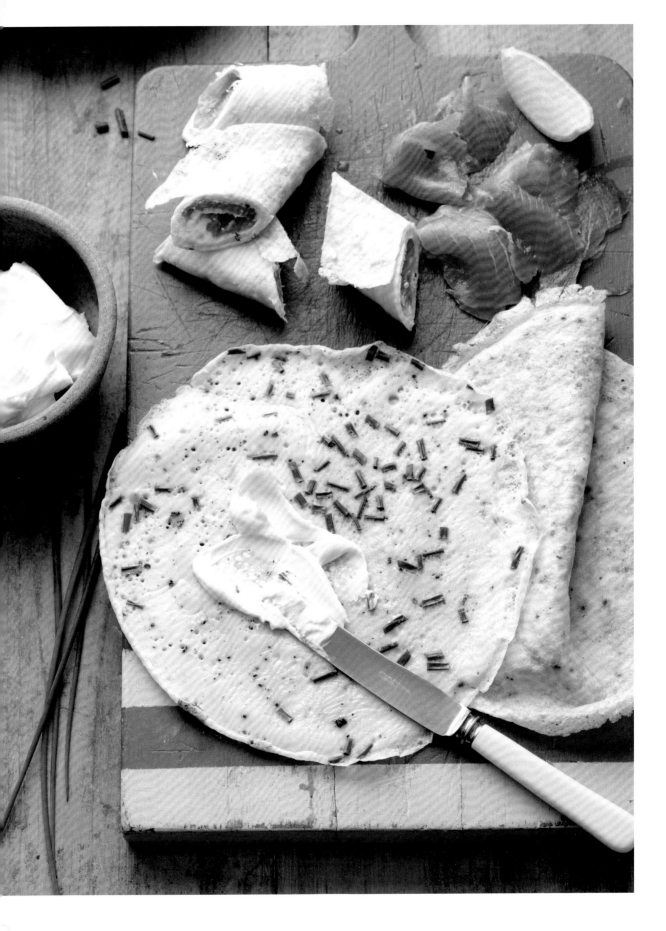

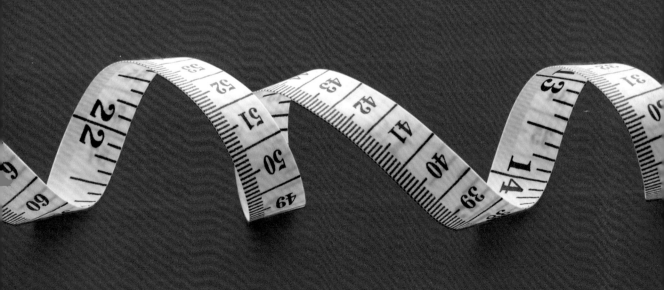

sweet
things

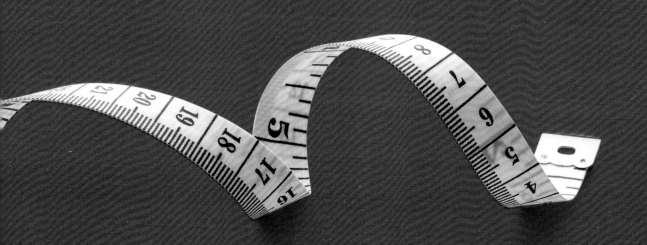

124
CALORIES
PER SERVING

french apple tarts

SERVES 6
PREP: 10 MINUTES
COOK: 15 MINUTES

320g ready-rolled sheet
   of light puff pastry
½ tbsp plain flour, for rolling
2 tbsp apricot jam
3 small eating apples
   (each about 90g)
1 tbsp caster sugar
½ tsp ground cinnamon

Open freeze the cooled,
baked tarts until solid. Stack
in a rigid freezer-proof
container, interleaving them
with baking parchment.
Reheat from frozen as the
recipe for 8–10 minutes.

**Light puff pastry is available in most major supermarkets
and contains 30% less fat than standard puff pastry. Rolling
the pastry even thinner makes more tarts containing fewer
calories.**

Preheat the oven to 220°C/Fan 200°C/Gas 7. Lightly dust
your work surface with flour and unroll the pastry onto it. Use
a rolling pin to roll out the pastry until it is very thin – around
3mm thick and long enough to cut out 6 x 11cm rounds.

Use an 11cm plain biscuit cutter or small saucer to cut out six
pastry discs. Place the discs on a large baking sheet lined with
parchment. Brush the centre of each disc thickly with apricot
jam using the back of a teaspoon.

Peel the apples and cut them into quarters. Remove the
cores and very thinly slice the apples. Arrange the apple slices
in concentric circles on each pastry disc. Mix the sugar and
cinnamon together and sprinkle them over the apples.

Bake for 12–15 minutes or until the pastry is puffed up and
golden brown and the apples are tender. Serve warm with
half-fat crème fraiche if you like.

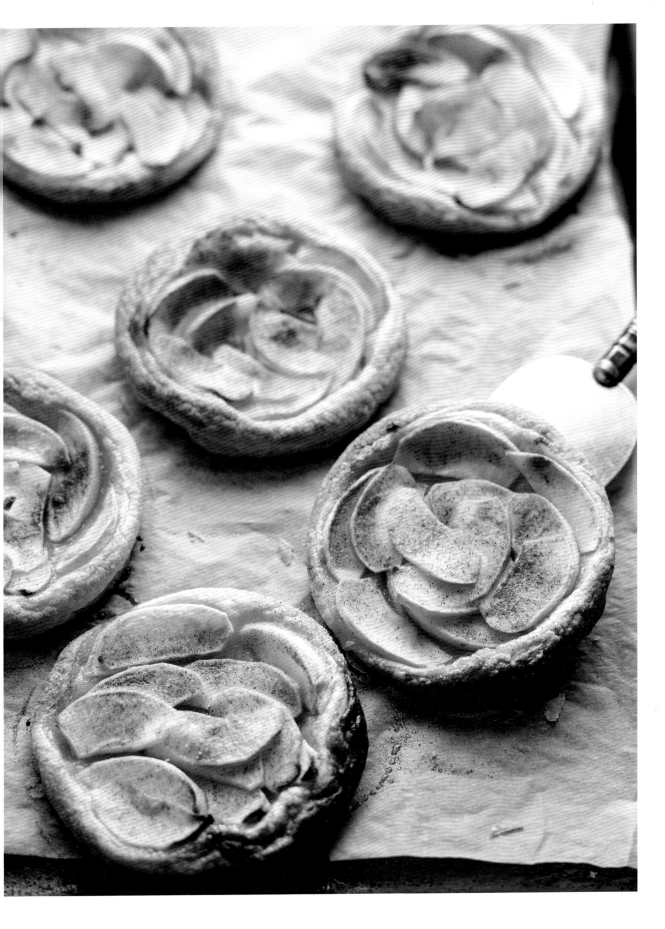

34
CALORIES
PER SERVING

strawberry granita

SERVES 4
PREP: 5 MINUTES,
PLUS FREEZING TIME

500g fresh strawberries
1 tbsp caster sugar
   (optional)

Tip: Slicing your strawberries before freezing means you can blitz them more quickly. It's a good idea to check that your blender is designed to crush ice or you could damage the blade and the crack the jug.

This super-low-calorie iced dessert is very quick to prepare as long as your fruit is already frozen. Either freeze your own, as I have done here, or buy bags of frozen fruit from the supermarket. It's important to use a sturdy blender designed to crush ice.

Put your freezer onto fast freeze or clear some space in the rapid freezing section at least an hour before preparing the strawberries.

Line a large baking tray with baking parchment. Hull the strawberries and cut them into slices. Spread the slices over a baking tray and freeze until solid. This should take 2–4 hours. Transfer the strawberries to a freezer bag and seal.

When you are ready to make the granita, put the frozen strawberries in a sturdy blender or food processor and blitz on the pulse setting into fine, strawberry ice granules. Add a little sugar if your strawberries don't have much flavour – some frozen fruit from the supermarket can be a little sour – and blitz again. Spoon into pretty glasses and serve.

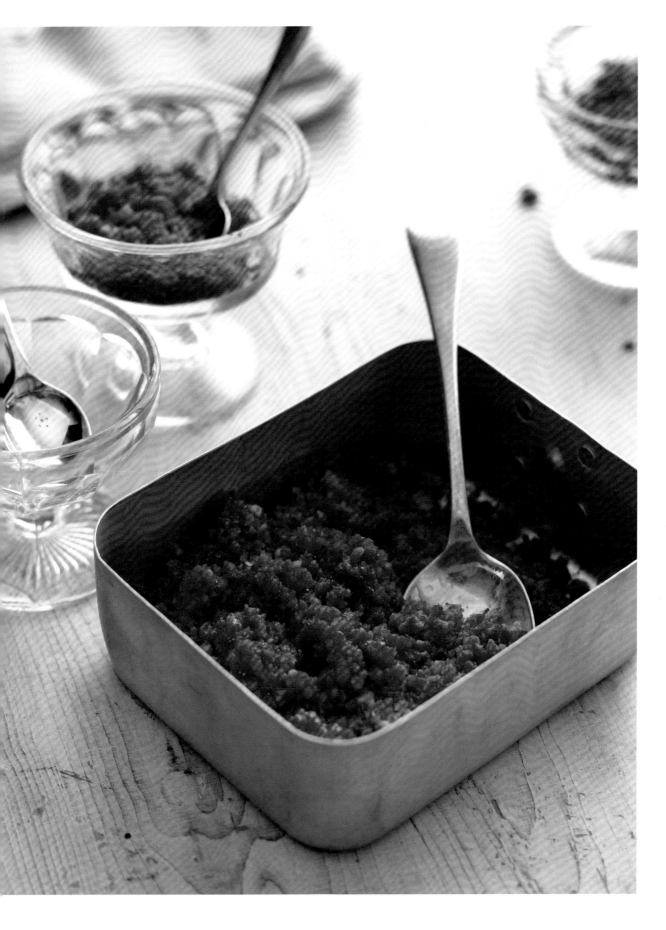

56
CALORIES
PER CAKE

lemon and poppy seed madeleines

MAKES 12

PREP: 5 MINUTES

COOK: 15 MINUTES

2 large eggs
50g caster sugar
finely grated zest
  of 2 lemons
1 tsp poppy seeds (optional)
75g plain flour
oil, for spraying or brushing

Freeze the madeleines individually by wrapping in foil and placing in a freezer bag. Freeze for up to 3 months. Unwrap while frozen and defrost at room temperature for about 30 minutes before serving.

Tip: Madeleine tins are available in cookshops, department stores and online. They are a worthwhile investment if you like baking but find the idea of portion control really useful.

I was inspired to make this cake after seeing tiny individual cakes being sold in my local supermarket. It got me thinking that we have all become so used to being served giant slabs of cake that we've forgotten that something small and delicate can be just as satisfying and a lot less sickly. Individual cakes can be wrapped in foil and frozen so you aren't tempted to eat too many at once. I sometimes serve madeleines with fresh raspberries and half-fat crème fraiche for a quick dessert.

Preheat the oven to 200°C/Fan 180°C/Gas 6.

Put the eggs, sugar, lemon zest and poppy seeds in a heatproof bowl and place over a pan of gently simmering water. Whisk using an electric whisk until the mixture is pale, creamy and thick enough to leave a trail when the whisk is lifted – this should take about 5 minutes.

Carefully remove the bowl from the heat and continue whisking for a further 1–2 minutes. Sift over half the flour and, using a large metal spoon, lightly fold the flour into the egg mixture. Sift over the remaining flour and fold in. It's important to use gentle movements to retain as much air as possible in the batter but you'll need to watch out for pockets of flour.

Carefully spoon the batter into a 12-hole non-stick madeleine tin that has been lightly sprayed or brushed with oil. Bake for 6–7 minutes until well risen, pale golden brown and firm to the touch. Allow to cool completely in the tin before gently removing them one at a time.

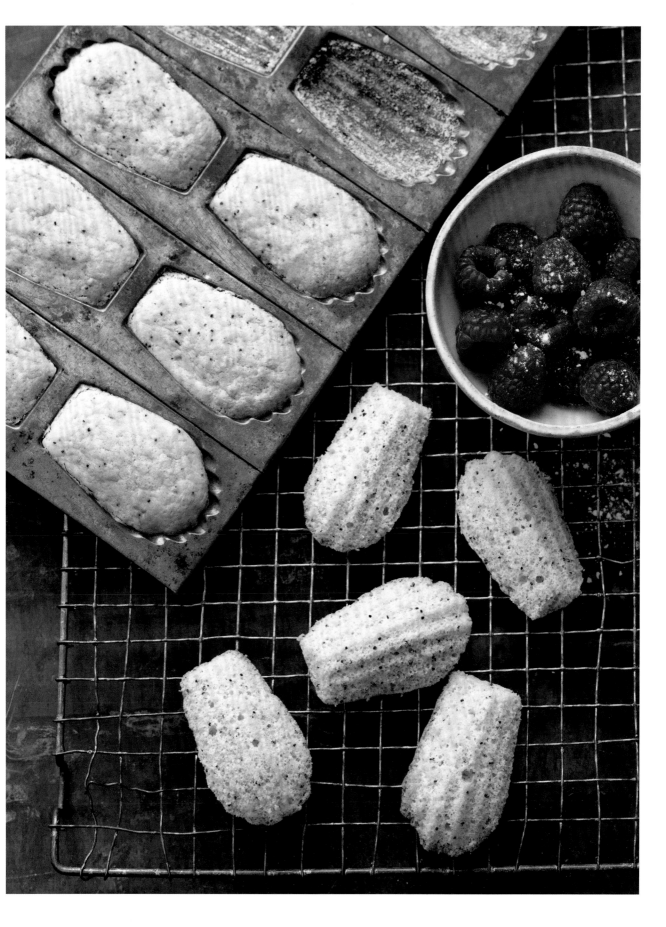

170
CALORIES
PER SERVING

strawberry shortcakes

SERVES 12

PREP: 15 MINUTES

COOK: 15 MINUTES

250g self-raising flour,
plus extra for rolling
40g butter, cubed and
fridge cold
1 tbsp caster sugar
125ml semi-skimmed milk,
plus extra for brushing
150ml whipping cream
400g fresh strawberries,
hulled and roughly
chopped
25g reduced-sugar
strawberry jam

Freeze the cooled, unfilled
scones in a freezer bag for
up to 3 months. To serve,
place the frozen scones on
a baking tray and reheat in a
preheated oven at 190°C/
Fan 170°C/Gas 5 for 6–8
minutes. Alternatively,
defrost the cooked scones
at room temperature for
30 minutes then warm them
in a microwave oven on full
power for 20–30 seconds.

Scones freeze incredibly well so it's always worth making
a big batch. Three scones will serve six people as each person
has just half a scone to keep the calories low. Top with a little
whipped cream and lots of fresh strawberries and no one will
notice. The quantities of strawberries and cream in this recipe
will top 12 scone halves, so you'll need to reduce the quantities
if you're preparing six at a time.

Preheat the oven to 220°C/Fan 200°C/Gas 7. Line a large
baking tray with baking parchment. Put the flour, butter and
sugar in a food processor and blitz on the pulse setting until
the mixture resembles breadcrumbs.

With the motor running, slowly add the milk and blend for
a few seconds more until the mixture comes together and
forms a light, spongy dough.

Turn the dough onto a well-floured surface and knead lightly
until smooth and soft. Roll with a rolling pin until it is around
2cm thick.

Using a 6cm plain biscuit cutter, cut four rounds from the
dough and place them on the prepared baking tray, spacing
them well apart. Knead again, then roll the trimmings and cut
two more rounds from the dough.

Brush just the top of the scones with a little milk and bake
in the centre of the oven for 15 minutes or until well risen and
golden brown. Remove the tray from the oven and set aside
to cool for a few minutes.

Whip the cream until soft peaks form. Mix the strawberries
with the strawberry jam. Cut the scones in half and top with
the strawberries and cream. Serve warm.

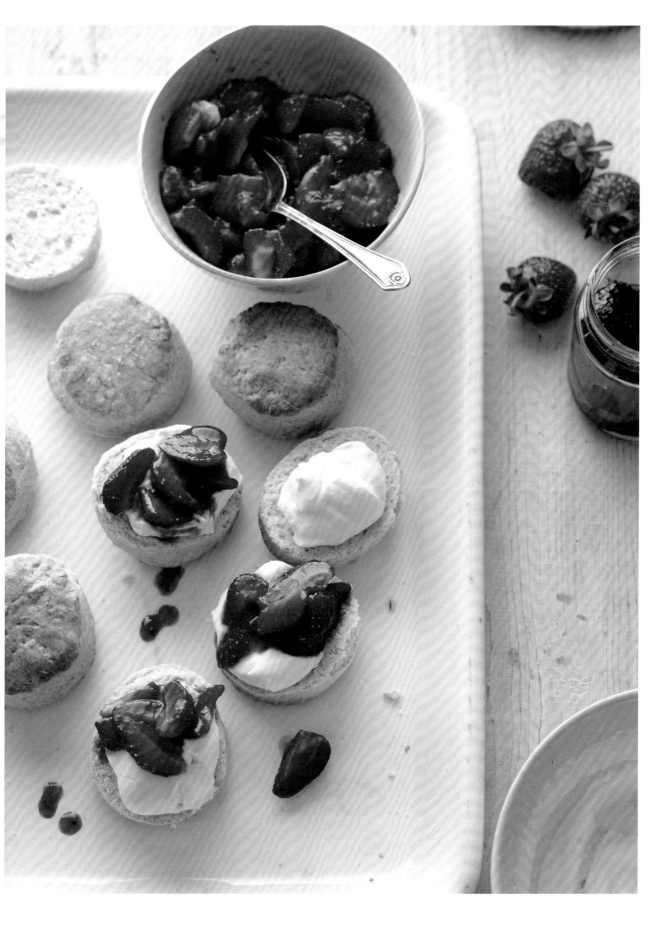

132
CALORIES
PER SERVING

apricot strudel

SERVES 6

PREP: 15 MINUTES

COOK: 20 MINUTES

3 filo pastry sheets
(each about 45g)
oil, for spraying or brushing
75g marzipan
411g can apricot halves
in juice
1 tbsp flaked almonds

Tip: Spray your grater lightly with oil to stop the marzipan sticking.

This simple strudel recipe uses canned apricot halves rather than apples, so it's very quick to cook. The marzipan adds flavour and sweetness. Your filo pastry will need to be around 45 x 25cm for this recipe. If it is a little narrower, stagger the sheets slightly as you lay them down. This won't be noticeable by the time you roll out the pastry.

Preheat the oven to 200°C/Fan 180°C/Gas 6. Place the filo sheets on a baking tray, lightly brushing or spraying them with oil between each sheet.

With one short side of the pastry pile facing you, coarsely grate the marzipan over the bottom two-thirds of the pastry, leaving a 5cm border at the bottom and both sides.

Drain the apricots in a sieve and roughly chop them on a board. Scatter the apricots over the marzipan. Fold up the bottom of the pastry until it begins to cover the marzipan, and then fold in the sides. Roll the strudel from the bottom gently but firmly to enclose the filling. Turn so the seal is at the bottom of the roll.

Spray the strudel lightly with oil and scatter the flaked almonds over the top. Bake for 20 minutes or until golden and crisp. Leave to cool for 10 minutes before cutting.

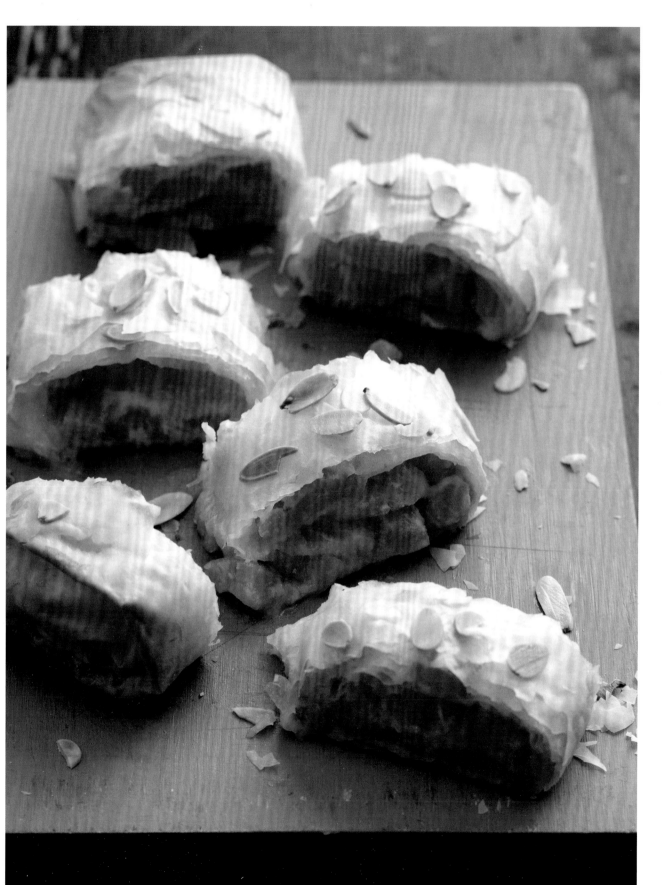

254
CALORIES
PER SERVING

ten-minute trifle

SERVES 6

PREP: 10 MINUTES

6 boudoir biscuits
(sponge fingers)
6 tbsp Marsala wine
or sweet sherry
415g can peach slices
in juice, drained,
reserving the juice
300ml low fat ready-made
custard (fresh if possible)
150g fresh or frozen
raspberries
150ml whipping cream,
well chilled
15g toasted flaked almonds
20g amaretti biscuits
(about 3)

Sometimes only something rich and creamy will do, and that's when these individual trifles really hit the spot. Whipping cream contains fewer calories than double cream and makes a lovely soft, billowy topping for the fruit.

Divide the boudoir biscuits between six dessert dishes or put them in a glass bowl. Spoon a tablespoon of Marsala or sweet sherry over each sponge, then 6 tablespoons of the reserved juice.

Spoon the custard on top of the sponge and top with peach slices and raspberries. Whip the cream with an electric whisk until soft and billowy. Spoon the whipped cream on top of the fruit.

Scatter with flaked toasted almonds and crush the amaretti biscuits with your fingers then sprinkle them over the top. Serve immediately.

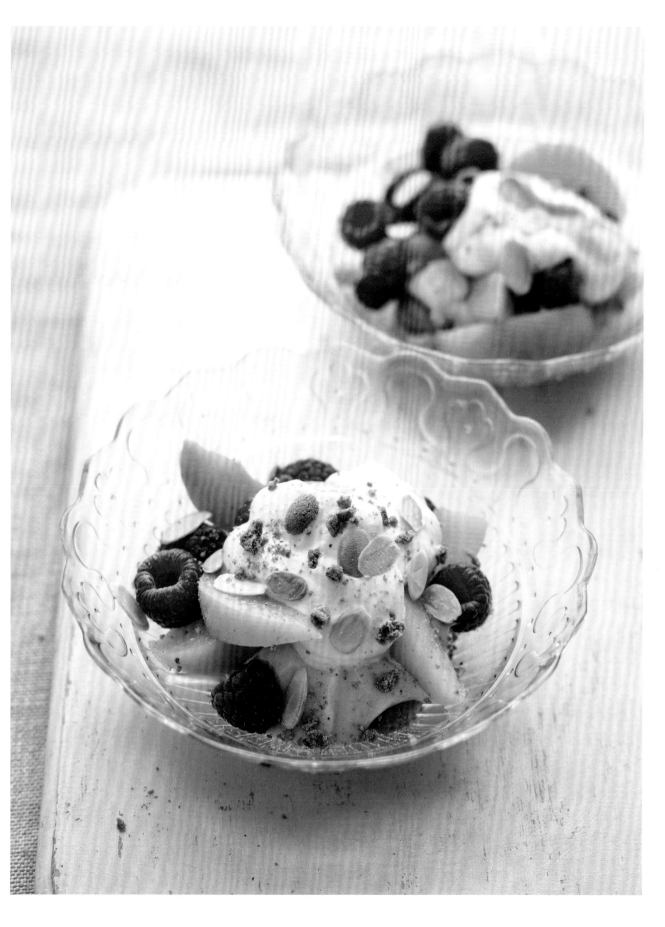

183
CALORIES
PER SERVING

chocolate orange pears

SERVES 4

PREP: 5 MINUTES

COOK: 15 MINUTES

1 large orange
50g caster sugar
1 cinnamon stick
4 firm but ripe pears
50g plain, dark chocolate
   (about 70% cocoa)

Poached pears make a popular dessert, especially when combined with dark chocolate. They are lovely served warm after a winter weekend lunch and the pears are also delicious eaten cold at breakfast with spoonfuls of low-fat natural yoghurt or quark.

Peel the orange rind into long strips with a potato peeler and put it into a saucepan. Add the sugar and cinnamon stick. Cut the orange in half and squeeze out the juice. Pour the juice into the saucepan.

Peel the pears, cut them in half and place them in the saucepan. Add enough cold water to cover and bring to a simmer. Cook for 15 minutes or until tender. Meanwhile, melt the chocolate in a heatproof bowl over a pan of gently simmering water (or in the microwave) until smooth.

Drain the pears and divide them between four dishes. Drizzle the hot chocolate over the pears and serve.

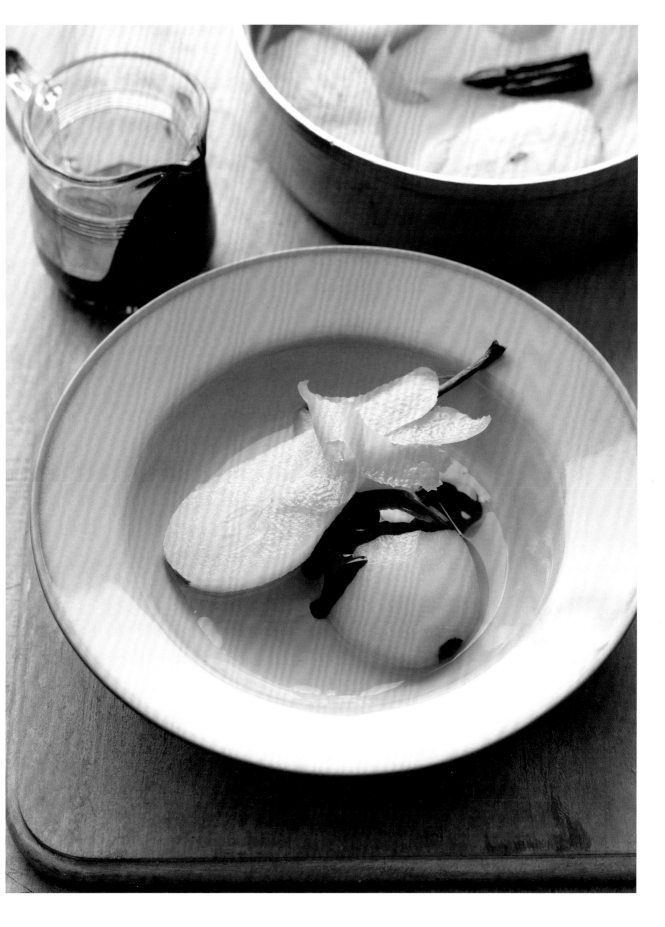

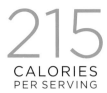

215
CALORIES
PER SERVING

lime and ginger
mini cheesecakes

SERVES 6

**PREP: 10 MINUTES,
PLUS CHILLING**

6 gingernut biscuits
finely grated zest of 2 limes
(about 1 tbsp)
250g quark, well chilled
and drained
25g caster sugar
150ml double cream,
well chilled
100g fresh raspberries
(optional)

Quark is a naturally low-fat soft cheese and is brilliant for when you want creaminess without the calories. These little cheesecakes contain just enough double cream to taste rich and luxurious and are a doddle to prepare.

Take six ramekins or pretty glasses and crumble one ginger biscuit into the base of each.

Reserve a little lime zest for decoration and lightly mix the rest with the quark and caster sugar. Whip the cream in a small bowl until soft peaks form and fold it into the quark mixture.

Spoon the mixture onto the ginger biscuit base and decorate with lime zest and fresh raspberries if you like. Cover with cling film and chill for at least 30 minutes before serving.

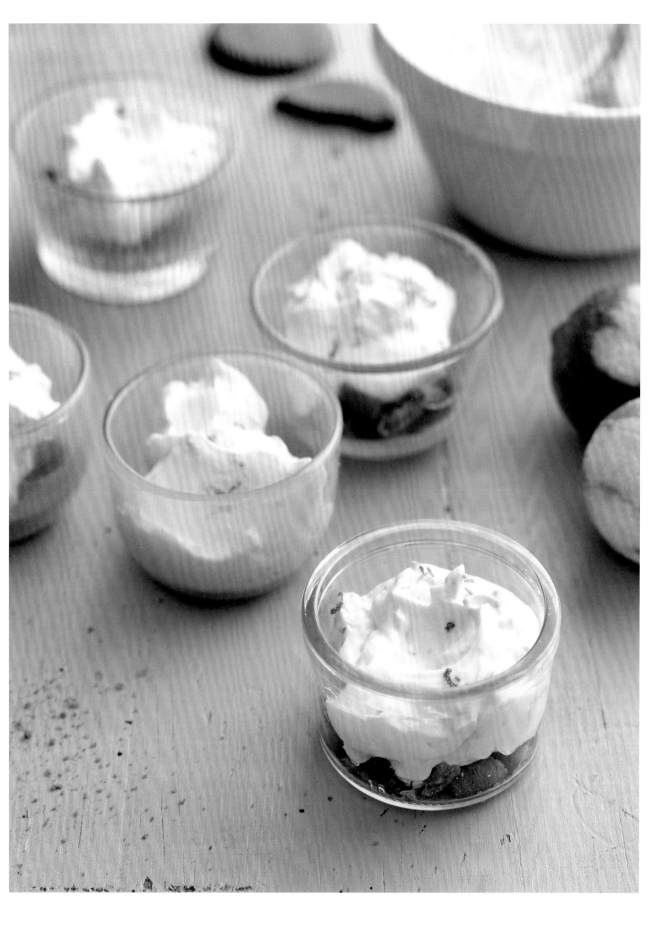

iced fruit sticks

SERVES 6
PREP: 15 MINUTES,
PLUS FREEZING TIME

½ small pineapple
(about 500g)
250g small strawberries,
hulled
150g large seedless grapes,
picked off the vine
short skewers or lolly sticks
chocolate sauce (see right),
for serving

These are my version of fruit ice lollies and a secret weapon against snacking. Keeping frozen fruit in the freezer means there is never an excuse to get out the ice cream instead. Threading the fruit onto skewers makes simple lollies that can be served as a snack or even a dessert with a hot chocolate sauce for dipping.

Put your freezer onto fast freeze or clear some space in the rapid freezing section at least an hour before preparing the fruit.

Put the pineapple on a board and cut off the top and bottom. Carefully cut off all the coarse skin, then use the tip of a knife to pick out and discard any prickly 'eyes'.

Cut the pineapple in half lengthways and then in half again. Remove the central core as it can be quite tough.

Cut the pineapple into chunky pieces and thread it with the other fruit onto short skewers. Place the skewers on a baking tray lined with baking parchment. Freeze until solid, then pack into a freezer-proof container, cover and freeze for up to 1 month.

Take out of the freezer and stand at room temperature for 5–10 minutes before eating – just enough time for them to soften enough to eat easily. (They will still be extremely cold, so watch out if you have sensitive teeth.)

Chocolate sauce: Break 50g plain dark chocolate (about 70% cocoa) into a heatproof bowl and melt in the microwave or over a pan of simmering water until smooth. Allow to cool slightly before serving as a dip for the fruit sticks. Serves 6. Calories per serving: 42

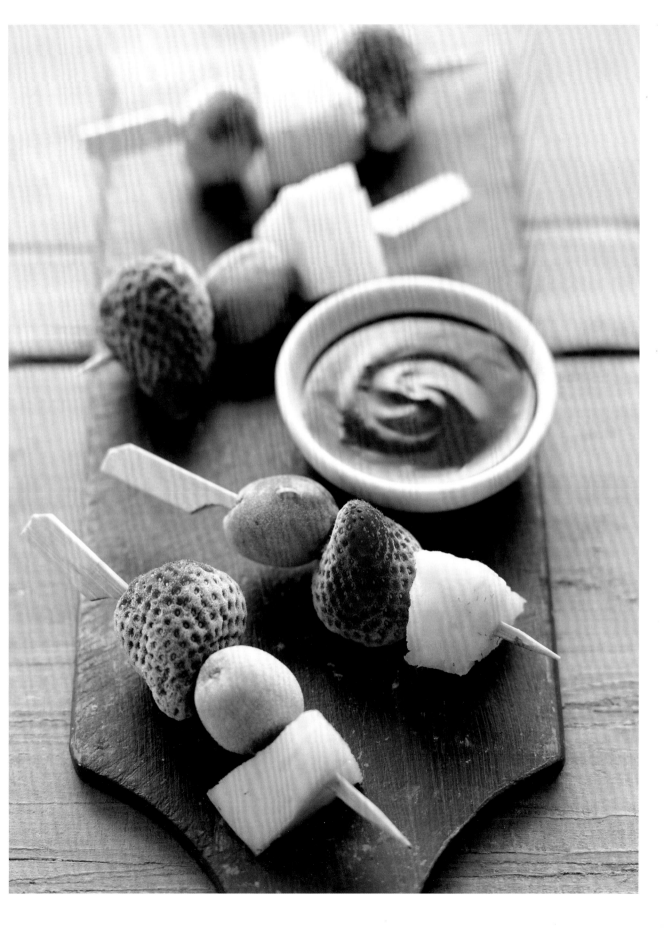

69
CALORIES
PER SERVING

mango and passion fruit fool

SERVES 4
PREP: 10 MINUTES

1 large, fresh ripe mango
   (about 315g)
200g fat-free Greek-
   style yoghurt
1 tsp caster sugar
½ tsp vanilla bean paste
   or vanilla extract
1 passion fruit

Tip: Vanilla bean paste can be found in major supermarkets and online and saves the hassle of splitting and scraping whole vanilla pods. It contains vanilla seeds that make the yoghurt taste sweeter without the need for lots of sugar.

A super-quick dessert that will keep well in the fridge for a couple of days. A ripe mango is naturally sweet, so there is no need to add extra sugar to the purée.

Cut the mango in half on either side of the large flat stone. Using a serving spoon, scoop the mango flesh away from the skin and put in a food processor or blender. (You should have around 180g flesh.) Remove the skin from the sides of the stones and carefully strip off the remaining mango flesh. Add to the rest.

Blitz the mango to a smooth purée. You may need to remove the lid and push the mixture down a couple of times with a rubber spatula until you achieve the right consistency.

Mix the yoghurt with the sugar and vanilla. Stir in roughly a third of the mango purée. Spoon alternate layers of mango purée and mango yoghurt into four glass dishes or tumblers. Swirl lightly with the tip of a knife.

Cut the passion fruit in half and scoop a little of the pulp onto each of the puddings. Cover and chill if not serving immediately.

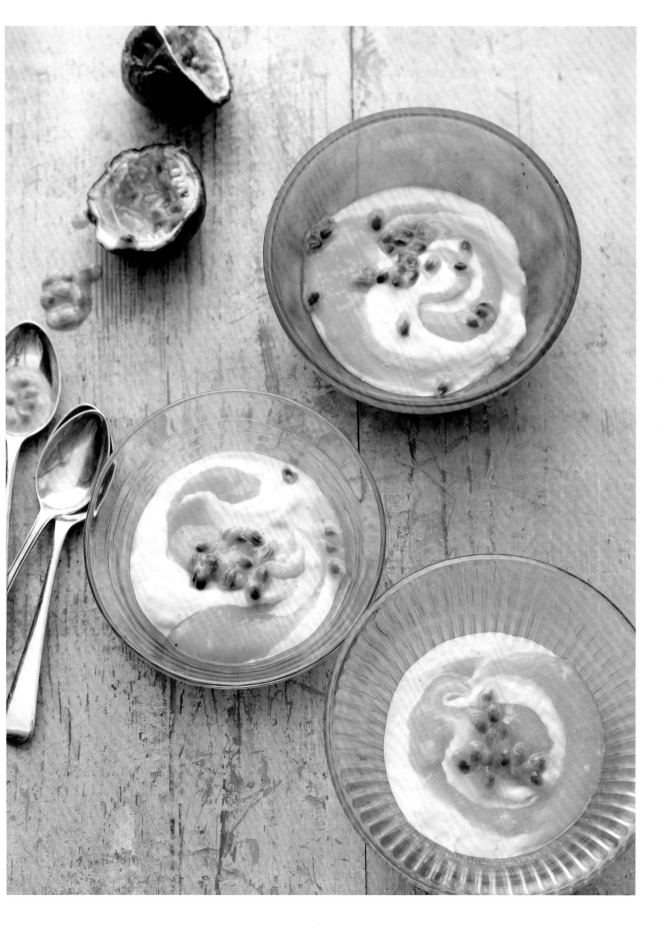

a few notes on the recipes

INGREDIENTS

Where possible, choose free-range chicken, meat and eggs. Eggs used in the recipes are medium unless otherwise stated.

All poultry and meat has been trimmed of as much hard or visible fat as possible, although there may be some marbling within the meat. Boneless, skinless chicken breasts weigh around 175g. Fish has been scaled, gutted and pin-boned, and large prawns are deveined. You'll be able to buy most fish and seafood ready prepared but ask your fishmonger if not and they will be happy to help.

PREPARATION

Do as much preparation as possible before you start to cook. Discard any damaged bits, and wipe or wash fresh produce before preparation unless it's going to be peeled.

Onions, garlic and shallots are peeled unless otherwise stated, and vegetables are trimmed. Lemons, limes and oranges should be well washed before the zest is grated. Weigh fresh herbs in a bunch, then trim off the stalks before chopping the leaves. I've used medium-sized vegetables unless stated. As a rule of thumb, a medium-sized onion and potato (such as Maris Piper) weighs about 150g.

All chopped and sliced meat, poultry, fish and vegetable sizes are approximate. Don't worry if your pieces are a bit larger or smaller than indicated, but try to keep to roughly the size so the cooking times are accurate. Even-sized pieces will cook at the same rate, which is especially important for meat and fish.

I love using fresh herbs in my recipes, but you can substitute frozen herbs in most cases. Dried herbs will give a different, more intense flavour, so use them sparingly.

The recipes have been tested using sunflower oil, but you can substitute vegetable, groundnut or mild olive oil. I use dark soy sauce in the test kitchen but it's fine to use light instead – it'll give a milder flavour.

CALORIE COUNTS

Nutritional information does not include the optional serving suggestions. When shopping, you may see calories described as kilocalories on food labels; they are the same thing.

HOW TO FREEZE

Freezing food will save you time and money, and lots of the dishes in this book freeze extremely well. If you don't need all the servings at the same time, freeze the rest for another day. Where there are no instructions for freezing a dish, freezing won't give the best results once reheated.

When freezing food, it's important to cool it rapidly after cooking. Separate what you want to freeze from what you're going to serve and place it in a shallow, freezer-proof container. The shallower the container, the quicker the food will cool (putting it in the freezer while it's still warm will raise the freezer temperature and could affect other foods). Cover loosely, then freeze as soon as it's cool.

If you're freezing a lot of food at once, for example after a bulk cooking session or a big shop, flip the fast freeze button on at least two hours before adding the new dishes and leave it on for twenty-four hours afterwards. This will reduce the temperature of your freezer and help ensure that food is frozen as rapidly as possible.

When freezing food, expel as much air as possible by wrapping it tightly in a freezer bag or foil to help prevent icy patches, freezer burn and discolouration, or flavour transfer between dishes. Liquids expand when frozen, so leave a 4–5cm gap at the top of containers.

If you have a small freezer and need to save space, flat-freeze thick soups, sauces and casseroles in strong zip-seal freezer bags. Fill the bag halfway, then turn it over and flatten it until it is around 1–2cm thick, pressing out as much air as possible and sealing firmly.

Place delicate foods such as breaded chicken or fish fillets and burgers on a tray lined with baking parchment, and freeze in a single layer until solid before placing in containers or freezer bags. This method is called open freezing and helps stop foods sticking together in a block, so you can grab what you need easily.

Label everything clearly, and add the date so you know when to eat it at its best. I aim to use food from the freezer within about four months.

DEFROSTING

For the best results, most foods should be defrosted slowly in the fridge for several hours or overnight. For safety's sake, do not thaw dishes at room temperature.

Flat-frozen foods (see above) will thaw and begin to reheat at almost the same time. Just rinse the bag under hot water and break the mixture into a wide-based pan. Add a dash of water and warm over a low heat until thawed. Increase the heat, adding a little more water if necessary, and simmer until piping hot throughout.

Ensure that any foods that have been frozen are thoroughly cooked or reheated before serving.

HOW TO GET THE BEST RESULTS
Measuring with spoons

Spoon measurements are level unless otherwise stated. Use a set of measuring spoons for the best results; they're endlessly useful, especially if you're watching your sugar, salt or fat intake.

1 tsp (1 teaspoon) = 5ml
1 dsp (1 dessertspoon) = 10ml
1 tbsp (1 tablespoon) = 15ml

A scant measure is just below level and a heaped measure is just above. An Australian tablespoon holds 20ml, so Australian cooks should use three level teaspoon measures instead.

CONVERSION CHARTS

Oven temperature guide

	Electricity °C	Electricity °F	Electricity (fan) °C	Gas Mark
Very cool	110	225	90	$1/4$
	120	250	100	$1/2$
Cool	140	275	120	1
	150	300	130	2
Moderate	160	325	140	3
	170	350	160	4
Moderately hot	190	375	170	5
	200	400	180	6
Hot	220	425	200	7
	230	450	210	8
Very hot	240	475	220	9

Liquid measurements

Metric	Imperial	Australian	US
25ml	1fl oz		
60ml	2fl oz	$1/4$ cup	$1/4$ cup
75ml	3fl oz		
100ml	$3\frac{1}{2}$fl oz		
120ml	4fl oz	$1/2$ cup	$1/2$ cup
150ml	5fl oz		
180ml	6fl oz	$3/4$ cup	$3/4$ cup
200ml	7fl oz		
250ml	9fl oz	1 cup	1 cup
300ml	$10\frac{1}{2}$fl oz	$1\frac{1}{4}$ cups	$1\frac{1}{4}$ cups
350ml	$12\frac{1}{2}$fl oz	$1\frac{1}{2}$ cups	$1\frac{1}{2}$ cups
400ml	14fl oz	$1\frac{3}{4}$ cups	$1\frac{3}{4}$ cups
450ml	16fl oz	2 cups	2 cups
600ml	1 pint	$2\frac{1}{2}$ cups	$2\frac{1}{2}$ cups
750ml	$1\frac{1}{4}$ pints	3 cups	3 cups
900ml	$1\frac{1}{2}$ pints	$3\frac{1}{2}$ cups	$3\frac{1}{2}$ cups
1 litre	$1\frac{3}{4}$ pints	1 quart or 4 cups	1 quart or 4 cups
1.2 litres	2 pints		
1.4 litres	$2\frac{1}{2}$ pints		
1.5 litres	$2\frac{3}{4}$ pints		
1.7 litres	3 pints		
2 litres	$3\frac{1}{2}$ pints		

essential extras

Here's my list of suggested 50–150 calorie foods that you can use to supplement the 123 Plan. All calories listed in this list are approximate; a few wayward calories here and there won't make a difference to your allowance. See page 6 for more information on essential extras and how they fit into the plan. I've also listed some 'free' vegetable ideas, of which you can eat as much as you like! Make sure your plate is half filled with vegetables or salad, or serve them in a large bowl on the side. Eating more greens will help fill you up and provide lots of extra nutrients in your diet. Your skin will look better and the weight should drop off.

50 CALORIES PER SERVING

30g (about 5) ready-to-eat dried apricots
15g (1 tbsp) light mayo
30g (2 tbsp) hummus
40g drained artichoke antipasti in oil
60g whole olives

4 fresh apricots
200g fresh blackberries
200g fresh blackcurrants
100g fresh cherries
2 clementines or satsumas
100g fresh figs
1/2 grapefruit
85g grapes
2 kiwis
100g fresh mango
200g melon
1 medium nectarine
1 medium orange
1 medium peach
1 medium pear
125g fresh pineapple
100g canned pineapple in juice
2 plums
200g papaya
100g pomegranate seeds
200g raspberries
200g strawberries

100g fresh tomato salsa
50g tzatziki
1 level tbsp orange marmalade
1 level tbsp mango chutney
1 level tsp taramasalata
1 level tbsp honey

2cm slice (about 20g) ciabatta
1 x 10g rye crispbread, such as Ryvita
50g cooked puy lentils, green lentils
1 x measure (25ml) spirits (light or dark, e.g. rum, vodka)

1 tbsp single cream
1 tbsp half-fat crème fraiche
10g Parmesan
30g soft French goat's cheese
25g (1 1/2 tbsp) light soft cheese
150ml orange juice (not from concentrate)
100ml regular soy milk
100g low-fat natural yoghurt
50g (about 3 wafer thin slices) of ham, turkey or chicken

75 CALORIES PER SERVING

150ml semi-skimmed milk
100g low-fat cottage cheese
25g (small wedge) Camembert
1 tbsp double cream
1 tbsp crème fraiche
50g ricotta cheese
1/4 125g ball of fresh mozzarella

1/4 average avocado (35g)
50g smoked salmon
1 rasher back bacon, grilled or dry-fried
50g cooked, skinless chicken breast
100g cooked jumbo prawns (about 9)

1 medium apple
100g blueberries
25g dried mango

2 cream crackers
20g rice cakes (2 or 3)
20g plain breadsticks (about 4)
1/2 English muffin
1 slice medium white or brown bread
15g shop-bought (not takeaway) prawn crackers
1 oatcake

1/2 160g tin tuna in brine, drained
40g sun-dried (or sun-blush) tomatoes in oil, drained
30g (2 tbsp) raisins
1 medium egg, boiled

100 CALORIES PER SERVING

1 large egg
40g feta cheese
100g plain cottage cheese
50g (2½ tbsp) soured cream
25g blue cheese
100ml fresh custard
25g cooking chorizo
30g ready-to-eat chorizo
(about 5 thin slices)
25g salami (about 5 thin
slices)
1 heaped tbsp pesto

45g Parma ham
(about 3 slices)
30g smoked mackerel fillet
1 medium banana

1 level tbsp peanut butter
1 tbsp extra virgin olive oil
30g popping corn kernels
20g unsalted plain cashews
20g tortilla chips
25g wasabi peas

20g plain crisps

1 slice of thick cut bread
½ plain bagel
1 x 45g soft white bread roll
½ regular pitta bread
1 slice German style rye bread
1 crumpet
120g baked beans
45g dried couscous
30g dried wholewheat pasta
25g dried soba noodles
30g dried quinoa

125ml wine (white, red, rose)
125ml sparkling wine/
Champagne
½ pint lager
½ pint bitter
½ pint dry cider

150 CALORIES PER SERVING

35g Cheddar cheese
100g skinless chicken breast,
baked or grilled

100g cooked brown rice
115g cooked easy-cook white
rice
40g dried basmati rice
1 potato, baked, boiled or
mashed without fat
(195g raw weight)
130g baked sweet potato
(about ½ large potato)
40g dried rice noodles
50g dried egg noodles
100g cooked pasta
40g porridge oats
50g shop-bought naan bread
(about ½)

25g unsalted almonds
175ml wine (not sparkling)

'FREE' SAUCES

Brown sauce, in moderation;
each tbsp is 24 calories
Fish sauce (nam pla)
Ketchup, in moderation;
each tbsp is 20 calories
Horseradish sauce
Hot sauce (Tabasco)
Mint sauce (not jelly)
Mustard, any variety (English,
Dijon, wholegrain,
American)
Soy sauce
Vinegars (balsamic, white
wine, malt, etc.)
Worcestershire sauce

Any herbs or spices

'FREE' VEGETABLES

Artichokes, including tinned
hearts (but not in oil)
Asparagus
Aubergine
Baby sweetcorn
Beans, any green (not baked)
(French, runner, etc.)
Bean sprouts
Beetroot, fresh, cooked
or pickled
Broccoli
Brussels sprouts
Butternut squash
Cabbage, all kinds
(savoy, red, white)
Carrots
Cauliflower
Celeriac
Celery
Chicory
Chillies, including pickled
jalapeños
Cornichons
Courgettes
Cucumber
Fennel
Garlic
Kale
Leeks
Lemons
Limes
Lettuce and salad greens
(watercress, baby
spinach, romaine)
Mangetout
Marrow
Mushrooms
Onions
Peppers
Pickled onions
Radishes
Shallots
Spring onions
Sugar snap peas
Swede
Tomatoes, including tinned
(but not sun-dried)
Turnips

nutritional information
per serving

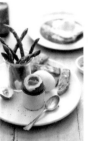

page 10 / serves 2
boiled eggs with asparagus soldiers

200/267*/193 energy (kcal)**
830/1116*/809** energy (kJ)
17.4/18.1*/11** protein (g)
2/16*/16.8** carb (g)
13.9/15*/9.6** fat (g)
3.8/4.5*/3.3** sat fat (g)
2.3/2.7*/2.8** fibre (g)
1.9/1.1*/1.1** sugars (g)
*toast soldiers/**on toast

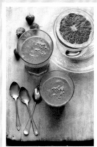

page 12 / serves 1
breakfast smoothie

261/32* energy (kcal)
1100/134* energy (kJ)
9.2/0.6* protein (g)
48.2/7.5* carb (g)
4.2/0.1* fat (g)
1.9/0* saturated fat (g)
5.0/1.4* fibre (g)
37.1/7.5* sugars (g)
*spiced grapefruit

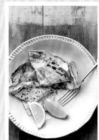

page 14 / serves 6
yoghurt pot pancakes

179 energy (kcal)
755 energy (kJ)
9.3 protein (g)
26.5 carbohydrate (g)
4.7 fat (g)
1.4 saturated fat (g)
1 fibre (g)
7.4 sugars (g)

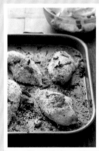

page 16 / serves 4
five minute nectarines

70 energy (kcal)
305 energy (kJ)
6.3 protein (g)
11.4 carbohydrate (g)
0.2 fat (g)
0 saturated fat (g)
1.2 fibre (g)
10.5 sugars (g)

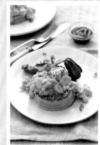

page 18 / serves 12
crushed berry layered yoghurt

102/143* energy (kcal)
434/601* energy (kJ)
6.5/2.9* protein (g)
19/22.7* carb (g)
0.4/4.2* fat (g)
0.2/2.3* sat fat (g)
3/2.7* fibre (g)
17.9/5.6* sugars (g)
*muesli

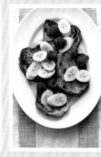

page 20 / serves 2
french toast with banana

447 energy (kcal)
1875 energy (kJ)
14.8 protein (g)
57.6 carbohydrate (g)
17.2 fat (g)
5.4 saturated fat (g)
4.5 fibre (g)
33.9 sugars (g)

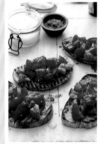

page 22 / serves 2
tomatoes on toasted sourdough

212 energy (kcal)
897 energy (kJ)
6.4 protein (g)
40.4 carbohydrate (g)
2.8 fat (g)
0.5 saturated fat (g)
3 fibre (g)
6 sugars (g)

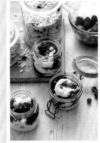

page 24 / serves 2
scrambled eggs with bacon

275 energy (kcal)
1140 energy (kJ)
18.8 protein (g)
0 carbohydrate (g)
22.2 fat (g)
8.3 saturated fat (g)
0 fibre (g)
0 sugars (g)

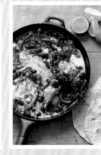

page 26 / serves 4
mexican breakfast

304 energy (kcal)
1281 energy (kJ)
18.5 protein (g)
37.8 carbohydrate (g)
9.8 fat (g)
3.3 saturated fat (g)
8.7 fibre (g)
10.4 sugars (g)

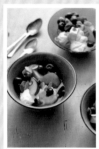

page 30 / serves 4
lemon and parmesan chicken

270/53* (kcal)
1140/220* energy (kJ)
46.6/1.8* protein (g)
7.8/3.7* carb (g)
4.9/3.5* fat (g)
1.9/0.6* sat fat (g)
0.3/2.3* fibre (g)
0.3/3.6* sugars (g)
*everyday salad

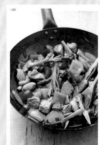

page 32 / serves 4
lemon chicken

230 energy (kcal)
971 energy (kJ)
35.4 protein (g)
11.2 carbohydrate (g)
5.2 fat (g)
1 saturated fat (g)
5.2 fibre (g)
8.6 sugars (g)

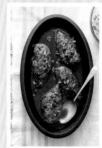

page 34 / serves 4
chicken with saffron, pistachios and honey

236 energy/118* (kcal)
998/501* energy (kJ)
42.9/4.1* protein (g)
7.1/24.2* carb (g)
4.0/0.2* fat (g)
0.8/0* saturated fat (g)
0.4/1.6* fibre (g)
6.1/0.1* sugars (g)
*coriander couscous

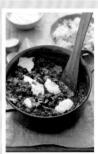

page 36 / serves 4
turkey chilli

323 energy (kcal)
1358 energy (kJ)
37.6 protein (g)
23.4 carbohydrate (g)
9.4 fat (g)
3.9 saturated fat (g)
7.3 fibre (g)
9.4 sugars (g)

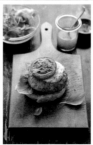

page 38 / serves 4
mediterranean turkey burgers

384 energy (kcal)
1621 energy (kJ)
45 protein (g)
30.7 carbohydrate (g)
9.7 fat (g)
3.8 saturated fat (g)
4.1 fibre (g)
5.8 sugars (g)

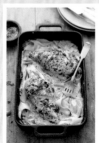

page 40 / serves 2
breton chicken

293 energy (kcal)
1232 energy (kJ)
43.8 protein (g)
4.5 carbohydrate (g)
10.1 fat (g)
2.9 saturated fat (g)
2.5 fibre (g)
2.3 sugars (g)

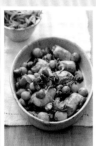

page 42 / serves 4
super-quick coq au vin

282 energy (kcal)
1187 energy (kJ)
42.0 protein (g)
3.5 carbohydrate (g)
9.4 fat (g)
2.4 saturated fat (g)
2.4 fibre (g)
3.4 sugars (g)

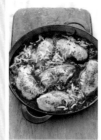

page 44 / serves 6
chicken parmiganna

253 energy (kcal)
1069 energy (kJ)
45.5 protein (g)
5.0 carbohydrate (g)
4.0 fat (g)
1.6 saturated fat (g)
1.3 fibre (g)
4.0 sugars (g)

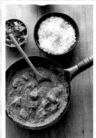

page 46 / serves 2
quick chicken curry

340 energy (kcal)
1433 energy (kJ)
49 protein (g)
21.6 carbohydrate (g)
6.9 fat (g)
1.0 saturated fat (g)
2.8 fibre (g)
16.0 sugars (g)

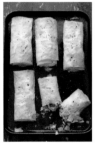

page 48 / serves 6
chicken and ham parcels

316 energy (kcal)
1332 energy (kJ)
30.3 protein (g)
26.5 carbohydrate (g)
9.8 fat (g)
4.5 saturated fat (g)
0.2 fibre (g)
1.5 sugars (g)

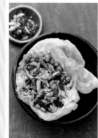

page 50 / serves 4
turkey lettuce wraps

158 energy (kcal)
665 energy (kJ)
29.8 protein (g)
3.5 carbohydrate (g)
2.8 fat (g)
0.7 saturated fat (g)
1.2 fibre (g)
3.0 sugars (g)

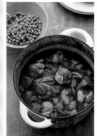

page 52 / serves 6
cheat's chicken casserole

256 energy (kcal)
1077 energy (kJ)
38.6 protein (g)
7.3 carbohydrate (g)
6.0 fat (g)
1.6 saturated fat (g)
3.3 fibre (g)
6.1 sugars (g)

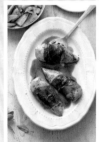

page 54 / serves 4
martini chicken

260/66* energy (kcal)
1097/274* energy (kJ)
46.1/1.0* protein (g)
4.0/7.6* carb (g)
4.2/3.7* fat (g)
1.2/2.1* saturated fat (g)
0/4.2* fibre (g)
4.0/7.1* sugars (g)
*lemon and parsley carrots

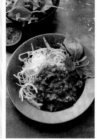

page 56 / serves 6
turkey bolognese

181/68* energy (kcal)
763/282* energy (kJ)
23.6/3.5* protein (g)
12.1/12.5* carb (g)
3.1/.5* fat (g)
0.5/0* saturated fat (g)
3.8/7* fibre (g)
8.3/12.2* sugars (g)
*cheat's spaghetti

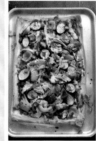

page 58 / serves 4
tex mex chicken tart

275 energy (kcal)
1156 energy (kJ)
17 protein (g)
35.1 carbohydrate (g)
7.2 fat (g)
2.4 saturated fat (g)
3.2 fibre (g)
6.6 sugars (g)

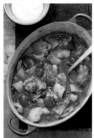

page 60 / serves 6
tom's paprika chicken

257 energy (kcal)
1080 energy (kJ)
36.9 protein (g)
9.7 carbohydrate (g)
6.9 fat (g)
1.6 saturated fat (g)
3.2 fibre (g)
8.2 sugars (g)

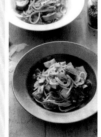

page 64 / serves 4
spaghetti on fire

256 energy (kcal)
1085 energy (kJ)
13.5 protein (g)
45.7 carbohydrate (g)
3.4 fat (g)
0.8 saturated fat (g)
6.5 fibre (g)
13.1 sugars (g)

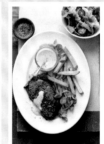

page 66 / serves 4
sirloin steak, chips and béarnaise sauce

516 energy (kcal)
2160 energy (kJ)
52.9 protein (g)
27 carbohydrate (g)
21.5 fat (g)
8.7 saturated fat (g)
1.6 fibre (g)
3.2 sugars (g)

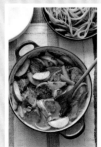

page 68 / serves 4
somerset pork and apples

298 energy (kcal)
1249 energy (kJ)
28.2 protein (g)
14.7 carbohydrate (g)
12.7 fat (g)
5.2 saturated fat (g)
1.7 fibre (g)
10 sugars (g)

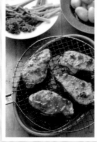

page 70 / serves 4
spiced mango pork steaks

241 energy (kcal)
1014 energy (kJ)
34.9 protein (g)
5.0 carbohydrate (g)
9.2 fat (g)
2.6 saturated fat (g)
0 fibre (g)
4.6 sugars (g)

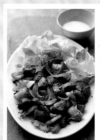

page 72 / serves 4
skewerless lamb kebabs

286 energy (kcal)
1196 energy (kJ)
28.7 protein (g)
13.7 carbohydrate (g)
13.3 fat (g)
4.8 saturated fat (g)
3.9 fibre (g)
11.5 sugars (g)

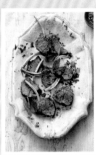

page 74 / serves 4
lamb cutlets with gremolata

334 energy (kcal)
1392 energy (kJ)
36.8 protein (g)
0.6 carbohydrate (g)
20.5 fat (g)
7.0 saturated fat (g)
0.4 fibre (g)
0.1 sugars (g)

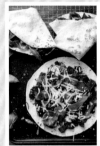

page 76 / serves 4
quick calzone

245 energy (kcal)
1036 energy (kJ)
12.5 protein (g)
40.3 carbohydrate (g)
4.8 fat (g)
2.3 saturated fat (g)
3.1 fibre (g)
4.6 sugars (g)

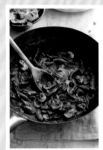

page 78 / serves 4
beef stroganoff

222 energy (kcal)
926 energy (kJ)
26.1 protein (g)
8.6 carbohydrate (g)
9.4 fat (g)
3.5 saturated fat (g)
2.4 fibre (g)
4.7 sugars (g)

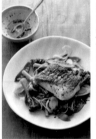

page 80 / serves 2
balsamic steak

227/199* energy (kcal)
948/842* energy (kJ)
32.8/14.2* protein (g)
0.3/31.3* carb (g)
10.1/2.7* fat (g)
4.3/0.5* sat fat (g)
0.7/14.7* fibre (g)
0.2/2.6* sugars (g)
*white bean mash

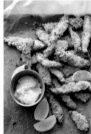

page 82 / serves 4
mozzarella meatballs lasagne

449 energy (kcal)
1883 energy (kJ)
33 protein (g)
32.7 carbohydrate (g)
18.9 fat (g)
8.4 saturated fat (g)
3.8 fibre (g)
11.0 sugars (g)

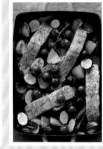

page 86 / serves 4
salmon provençal

308 energy (kcal)
1286 energy (kJ)
28 protein (g)
10.6 carbohydrate (g)
17.3 fat (g)
2.9 saturated fat (g)
3.9 fibre (g)
9.3 sugars (g)

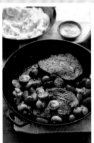

page 88 / serves 2
pan-fried cod with asian dressing

199 energy (kcal)
838 energy (kJ)
33.2 protein (g)
10.9 carbohydrate (g)
2.7 fat (g)
0.4 saturated fat (g)
5.5 fibre (g)
9.4 sugars (g)

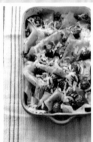

page 90 / serves 4
fish sticks

238/52* energy (kcal)
1007/215* energy (kJ)
26.1/1.0* protein (g)
24.5/2.5* carb (g)
4.6/4.2* fat (g)
0.8/0.6* sat fat (g)
0.3/0* fibre (g)
1.3/1.9* sugars (g)
*lemony garlic mayo

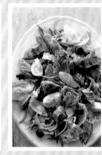

page 92 / serves 4
fresh tuna nicoise

283 energy (kcal)
1180 energy (kJ)
27.6 protein (g)
6.5 carbohydrate (g)
16.4 fat (g)
3.7 saturated fat (g)
3.9 fibre (g)
5.5 sugars (g)

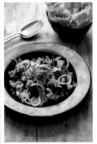

page 94 / serves 4
tuna and bean salad

139 energy (kcal)
587 energy (kJ)
19.3 protein (g)
13.7 carbohydrate (g)
1.0 fat (g)
0.2 saturated fat (g)
1.6 fibre (g)
3.9 sugars (g)

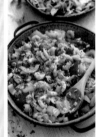

page 96 / serves 5
spanish prawns with rice

302 energy (kcal)
1276 energy (kJ)
23.4 protein (g)
38.4 carbohydrate (g)
7.2 fat (g)
2.5 saturated fat (g)
3.0 fibre (g)
6.7 sugars (g)

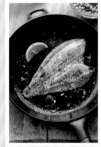

page 98 / serves 2
spicy seasoned fish

140 energy (kcal)
593 energy (kJ)
21.8 protein (g)
7.8 carbohydrate (g)
2.6 fat (g)
0.4 saturated fat (g)
0.4 fibre (g)
0.1 sugars (g)

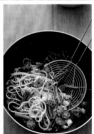

page 100 / serves 2
chilli lemon prawns with tomato and broccoli spaghetti

285 energy (kcal)
1207 energy (kJ)
31.3 protein (g)
32.7 carbohydrate (g)
4.1 fat (g)
0.7 saturated fat (g)
5.2 fibre (g)
4.2 sugars (g)

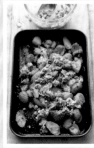

page 102 / serves 4
tuna and sweetcorn cheat's jackets

206 energy (kcal)
870 energy (kJ)
10.7 protein (g)
32.3 carbohydrate (g)
4.6 fat (g)
0.8 saturated fat (g)
2.6 fibre (g)
6.4 sugars (g)

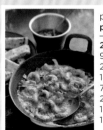

page 104 / serves 4
prawn korma

225 energy (kcal)
945 energy (kJ)
25.5 protein (g)
14.8 carbohydrate (g)
7.4 fat (g)
2.9 saturated fat (g)
1.4 fibre (g)
11.7 sugars (g)

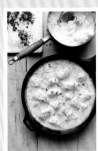

page 106 / serves 4
fast cod in parsley sauce

160/130* energy (kcal)
676/549* energy (kJ)
29.9/3.2* protein (g)
5.2/22.5* carb (g)
2.3/3.7* fat (g)
0.9/2.2* sat fat (g)
0.2/2.2* fibre (g)
3.3/1.7* sugars (g)
*mashed potatoes

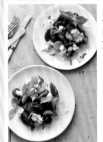

page 110 / serves 2
tomato, ricotta and basil salad

126 energy (kcal)
526 energy (kJ)
5.8 protein (g)
5.8 carbohydrate (g)
9.0 fat (g)
4.0 saturated fat (g)
2.0 fibre (g)
5.7 sugars (g)

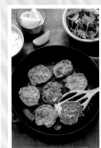

page 112 / serves 2
spiced courgette fritters

198 energy (kcal)
825 energy (kJ)
12.2 protein (g)
15 carbohydrate (g)
10.2 fat (g)
4.7 saturated fat (g)
2.3 fibre (g)
3.5 sugars (g)

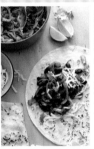

page 114 / serves 6
beany burritos

260 energy (kcal)
1104 energy (kJ)
11.3 protein (g)
49.2 carbohydrate (g)
3.4 fat (g)
1.5 saturated fat (g)
7.2 fibre (g)
7.5 sugars (g)

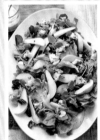

page 116 / serves 4
pear, blue cheese and walnut salad

130 energy (kcal)
541 energy (kJ)
4.8 protein (g)
6.9 carbohydrate (g)
9.4 fat (g)
3.6 saturated fat (g)
1.6 fibre (g)
6.9 sugars (g)

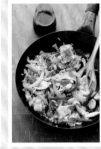

page 118 / serves 3
egg fried rice

251 energy (kcal)
1060 energy (kJ)
10.3 protein (g)
33.9 carbohydrate (g)
9.2 fat (g)
2.0 saturated fat (g)
4.6 fibre (g)
6.7 sugars (g)

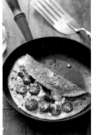

page 120 / serves 1
curried courgette omelette

313 energy (kcal)
1300 energy (kJ)
23.4 protein (g)
8.0 carbohydrate (g)
20.9 fat (g)
7.6 saturated fat (g)
4.3 fibre (g)
7.8 sugars (g)

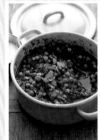

page 122 / serves 4
morroccan chickpea stew

246 energy (kcal)
1037 energy (kJ)
11.6 protein (g)
35.5 carbohydrate (g)
7.4 fat (g)
0.8 saturated fat (g)
9.3 fibre (g)
13 sugars (g)

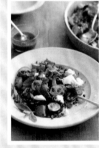

page 124 / serves 4
vegetable and goat's cheese salad

364/27* energy (kcal)
1529/112* energy (kJ)
16.5/0.5* protein (g)
42.9/2.4* carb (g)
14.9/1.7* fat (g)
7.5/0.3* sat fat (g)
9.3/1.0* fibre (g)
12.6/2.3* sugars (g)
*tomato dressing

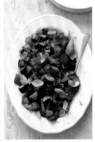

page 126 / serves 4
ratatouille

105 energy (kcal)
443 energy (kJ)
2.9 protein (g)
4.4 carbohydrate (g)
3.8 fat (g)
0.5 saturated fat (g)
6.3 fibre (g)
12.5 sugars (g)

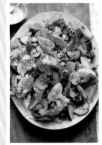

page 128 / serves 4
english garden egg salad

192 energy (kcal)
797 energy (kJ)
10.8 protein (g)
10.4 carbohydrate (g)
12.1 fat (g)
2.8 saturated fat (g)
4.4 fibre (g)
10.2 sugars (g)

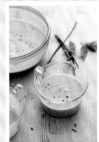

page 132 / serves 4
cooling cucumber and avocado soup

111 energy (kcal)
461 energy (kJ)
43 protein (g)
6.5 carbohydrate (g)
7.7 fat (g)
1.8 saturated fat (g)
2.4 fibre (g)
5.6 sugars (g)

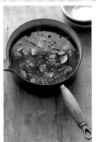

page 134 / serves 6
throw-it-together vegetable soup

67 energy (kcal)
280 energy (kJ)
3.5 protein (g)
10.1 carbohydrate (g)
1.6 fat (g)
0.3 saturated fat (g)
4.6 fibre (g)
7.8 sugars (g)

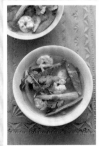

page 136 / serves 4
tom yum soup

89 energy (kcal)
374 energy (kJ)
13.6 protein (g)
3.9 carbohydrate (g)
2.1 fat (g)
0.4 saturated fat (g)
1.5 fibre (g)
2.2 sugars (g)

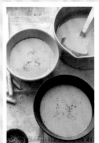

page 138 / serves 4
minted pea soup

89 energy (kcal)
375 energy (kJ)
7.4 protein (g)
13 carbohydrate (g)
1.2 fat (g)
0.3 saturated fat (g)
8.8 fibre (g)
4.1 sugars (g)

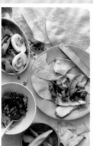

page 140 / serves 2
poppadum dippers

206/115* energy (kcal)
864/480* energy (kJ)
18.5/10.2* protein (g)
8.6/5.1* carb(g)
11/5.9* fat (g)
2.3/1.4* sat fat(g)
3.4/0.6* fibre (g)
3.2/0.5* sugars (g)
*egg and ham

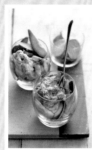

page 142 / serves 4
smoked trout pâté pot

142/124*/13 energy (kcal)**
598/515*/56** energy (kJ)
16.5/6.9*/0.5** protein (g)
10.4/3.1*/2.8** carb(g)
4.1/9.4*/0.1** fat (g)
1.4/1.9*/0** sat fat (g)
0.7/1.7*/0.2** fibre (g)
2.1/2.2*/0.1** sugars (g)
*avocado prawn pot
**french bread toasts

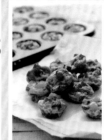

page 144 / serves 6
frittata bites

112 energy (kcal)
460 energy (kJ)
6.4 protein (g)
5.2 carbohydrate (g)
7.2 fat (g)
2.0 saturated fat (g)
1.6 fibre (g)
4.4 sugars (g)

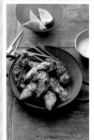

page 146 / serves 4
chicken tikka strips

99/110*/87 energy (kcal)**
418/461*/370** energy (kJ)
20.4/19.4*/19.6** protein (g)
1.5/0.4*/0.2** carb (g)
1.2/3.1*/0.9** fat (g)
0.3/0.6*/0.2** sat fat (g)
0.3/0.3*/0** fibre (g)
1.3/0.4*/0.2** sugars (g)
*tomato and pesto
**lemon and coriander

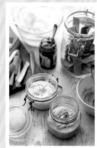

page 148 / serves 6
harissa hummus

42/92*/51 energy (kcal)**
178/381*/217** energy (kJ)
2.6/1.8*/1.8** protein (g)
3.0/1.4*/11** carb (g)
2.3/8.8*/0.3** fat (g)
0.3/0.7*/0** sat fat (g)
0.5/0*/0.5** fibre (g)
1.1/0.7*/0.6** sugars (g)
*taramasalata
**pitta dippers

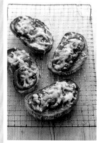

page 150 / serves 4
grilled tomatoes and cheese on toast

103 energy (kcal)
436 energy (kJ)
5.0 protein (g)
15.2 carbohydrate (g)
2.5 fat (g)
1.4 saturated fat (g)
1.4 fibre (g)
2.8 sugars (g)

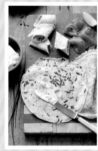

page 152 / serves 1
salmon and cream cheese snack rolls

158 energy (kcal)
660 energy (kJ)
15.3 protein (g)
0.7 carbohydrate (g)
10.5 fat (g)
3.2 saturated fat (g)
0 fibre (g)
0.7 sugars (g)

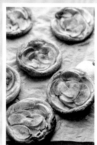

page 156 / serves 6
french apple tarts

124 energy (kcal)
524 energy (kJ)
1.9 protein (g)
20.6 carbohydrate (g)
4.2 fat (g)
2.1 saturated fat (g)
1.0 fibre (g)
10 sugars (g)

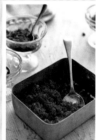

page 158 / serves 4
strawberry granita

34 energy (kcal)
141 energy (kJ)
1.0 protein (g)
7.5 carbohydrate (g)
0.1 fat (g)
0 saturated fat (g)
1.8 fibre (g)
7.5 sugars (g)

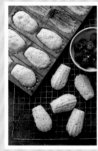

page 160 / makes 12
lemon and poppy seed madeleines

56 energy (kcal)
236 energy (kJ)
2.0 protein (g)
9.2 carbohydrate (g)
1.5 fat (g)
0.4 saturated fat (g)
0.3 fibre (g)
4.5 sugars (g)

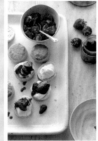

page 162 / serves 12
strawberry shortcakes

170 energy (kcal)
713 energy (kJ)
2.9 protein (g)
21.5 carbohydrate (g)
8.6 fat (g)
5.3 saturated fat (g)
1.4 fibre (g)
4.7 sugars (g)

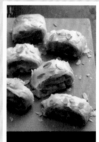

page 164 / serves 6
apricot strudel

132 energy (kcal)
560 energy (kJ)
2.8 protein (g)
23.5 carbohydrate (g)
3.2 fat (g)
0.3 saturated fat (g)
0.5 fibre (g)
11.9 sugars (g)

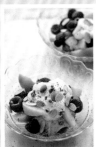

page 166 / serves 6
ten-minute trifle

254 energy (kcal)
1064 energy (kJ)
4.0 protein (g)
26.2 carbohydrate (g)
13.2 fat (g)
7.0 saturated fat (g)
1.6 fibre (g)
16.3 sugars (g)

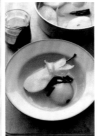

page 168/ serves 4
chocolate orange pears

183 energy (kcal)
774 energy (kJ)
1.3 protein (g)
38.6 carbohydrate (g)
3.6 fat (g)
2.1 saturated fat (g)
4.9 fibre (g)
38.5 sugars (g)

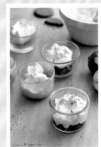

page 170 / serves 6
lime and ginger mini cheesecakes

215 energy (kcal)
895 energy (kJ)
7.0 protein (g)
14.4 carbohydrate (g)
14.7 fat (g)
10 saturated fat (g)
0 fibre (g)
10 sugars (g)

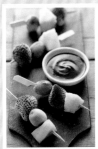

page 172 / serves 6
iced fruit sticks

60/42* energy (kcal)
258/178* energy (kJ)
0.8/0.4* protein (g)
14.8/5.3* carbohydrate (g)
0.2/2.3* fat (g)
0/1.4* saturated fat (g)
2.2/0.3* fibre (g)
14.8/5.2* sugars (g)
*chocolate sauce

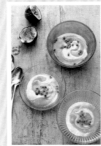

page 174 / serves 4
mango and passion fruit fool

69 energy (kcal)
298 energy (kJ)
5.6 protein (g)
12.1 carbohydrate (g)
0.2 fat (g)
0.1 saturated fat (g)
3.2 fibre (g)
3..3 sugars (g)

index

First published in Great Britain in 2015
by Orion Publishing Group Ltd
Carmelite House, 50 Victoria Embankment,
London EC4Y 0DZ
An Hachette UK Company

10 9 8 7 6 5

Text © Justine Pattison 2015
Design and layout © Orion 2015

A CIP catalogue record for this book is available
from the British Library.
ISBN: 978 1 4091 5471 6

Designer: Smith & Gilmour
Photographer: Cristian Barnett
Props stylist: Claire Bignell
Creative director: Justine Pattison
Nutritional analysis calculated by: Lauren Brignell
Recipe assistants: Kirsty Thomas, Vanessa Graham
Kitchen assistants: Jess Blain, Emily PB
Project editor: Jillian Young
Copy editor: Elise See Tai
Proofreader: Mary-Jane Wilkins
Indexer: Rosemary Dear

Printed and bound in Italy

*Every effort has been made to ensure that the
information in this book is accurate. The information
will be relevant to the majority of people but may not
be applicable in each individual case, so it is advised
that professional medical advice is obtained for
specific health matters. Neither the publisher nor
author accept any legal responsibility for any personal
injury or other damage or loss arising from the use or
misuse of the information in this book. Anyone making
a change in their diet should consult their GP,
especially if pregnant, infirm, elderly or under 16.*

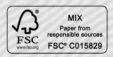

www.orionbooks.co.uk

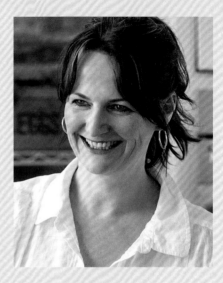

Acknowledgements

Firstly, huge thanks to everyone who enjoys my recipes
and the way I cook. You have given me such fantastic
feedback; I hope you like these dishes just as much.

I'm truly grateful to the very talented photographer
Cristian Barnett for wonderful photographs that really
make my food come to life. And the brilliant Claire
Bignell for her superb creative skills, selecting the
perfect props and helping make the recipes look
both beautiful and achievable.

Massive thanks to Lauren Brignell for all her invaluable
nutritional support and the hundreds of recipes she has
analysed over the past few months. Also, thanks to the
extremely hard-working Kirsty Thomas and Vanessa
Graham for carefully testing the recipes and assisting
on shoot days. Your skill and input has been invaluable.

At Orion, I would like to thank Amanda Harris for
believing in this project right from the beginning and
for trusting me to get on and develop the series. Also
thank you to Jillian Young, my fantastic editor, for her
guidance and professionalism and Helen Ewing for
her design support.

A big thank you to everyone at Smith & Gilmour for
making the books look eye-catching, practical and
readable. I'm also grateful to my agent, Zoe King, at
The Blair Partnership, for her constant encouragement
and enthusiasm.

And, a final thank you to my family and friends:
Angela, Ann, Angie, Bella, Charlotte, Clare, Emma,
Michelle, Rachel, Sarah and Tamsin for their
unwavering support.

Thank you to Kitchen Aid for kindly lending me
their brilliant mixers, blenders and food processors
for recipe testing.